Liberated from the Hill

Ruthenna Porterfield

To Devon
Thank you for your
support. Keep Dreaming
Yours

Liberated from the Hill

Ruthenna Porterfield

Printed in the United States of America
First Printing, 2021

ISBN 978-1-7359807-8-2

Publisher: Brittney Holmes Jackson & Co.
Stonecrest, GA 30038
www.BrittneyHolmesJackson.com

Dedication

For Jamal, Victoria and Oschare

Table of Contents

Preface

A in't nuthin' cross them tracks for us."

I heard this refrain often as a child growing up in my neighborhood. Liberty Hill boundaries were well defined in North Charleston, South Carolina. While East Montague Avenue was the four-lane thoroughfare connecting us to the rest of the city, the stoplight on the east end and the railroad tracks on the west, were like large signs saying, "This is the black part of town." The older residents deemed crossing the borders unnecessary. Everything you need was already on the hill. I wonder if that was the intention when the community was established, a century before I was born.

In 1864, Paul and Harriet Trescot owned 112 acres of farmland, north of Charleston. These "free persons of color" sold the land to four former slaves: Ishmael Grant, Aaron Middleton, and Plenty & William Lecque (Blakeney 2019). The goal was to establish a settlement for black men and their families with faith as the foundation. They donated one acre for the construction of St. Peter's African Methodist Episcopal Church on the southeast corner of the land, not far from where the stoplight is today. Then, they subdivided the remaining 111 acres into lots to be sold to recently freed blacks in 1871. One of those lots was sold to my Second Great-Grandfather, Guy E. Smalls. They named the area Liberty Hill to recognize the long-awaited freedom of the former slaves creating this new community (The Charleston Chronicle 2019).

The 'Liberty' part of my neighborhood's name was easy to understand. But where was the 'Hill?' There were no inclines on East Montague or any of the streets branching off on either side between the stoplight and the railroad tracks. From Sanders Avenue where St. Peter's still stands, to Gaynor Street, on the north side

1

where I lived, there was nothing to climb but little houses and tall trees. Yet, everything and everyone in the area was referred to as being 'on' or 'off' Liberty Hill. I figured the hill was a pinnacle; some point of pride to be reached by the people who lived there. If that is what those four free men were aspiring towards when they bought the land, they succeeded.

Liberty Hill was a self-sufficient community. By the 1980s, there was an elementary school and a high school. Good food could be found at several places. The shrimp dinners at Al's Diner were a staple. Momma Teen sold the best chilly bears on the south side of Montague; those little frozen cups of Kool-Aid were like heaven under the scorching sun. On the north side, kids lined up at Miss Mae's back door before and after school. She sold candy and snacks out of her kitchen. Grown folks danced and played pool at Ed Lee's little club. A few of them continued their evening at the Golden Dream Motel just a block east. St. Peter's AME was one of five churches dotting the streets. North Area Funeral Home sat at the neighborhood's west end. They helped lay many of our people to rest. You could raise your kids, bury your dead, have a little fun in between, and do it all without going past the stoplight or crossing the tracks. That is exactly what most of the residents of Liberty Hill did.

Felix Pinckney Center was the midpoint on that little stretch of Montague. There was a small park on the premises, as well as a community pool. Every summer, I went to the free lunch and Arts & Craft programs there. But our lunches were a little different. Along with the cold sandwiches in the gray paper trays provided by the city, kids were served hot fried chicken prepared by the grandmothers and aunts of Liberty Hill. We felt their love in every crispy, juicy thigh and drumstick browned to perfection. I always looked forward to the end of our Arts & Crafts program in July. Children displayed all the art they created during the last four weeks. The highlight was a show with a lip-sync and dance number by each age group.

When I was nine years old, I was chosen to be the lead in our age group's number for the finale. We chose Janet Jackson's *"What Have You Done for Me Lately."* I was so excited. The fact that I was the only girl with a Jheri Curl hairstyle long enough to play Janet, may have played a role in me getting the lead but I didn't care. I wanted to be out in front every year and this was my chance. It was like being one of the people I watched on the *Star Search* tv show every Saturday night. I secretly hoped my performance would make me famous. I wanted to look my best. A couple of hours before the show, I made the rookie mistake of purposefully wetting my Jheri Curl with water in hopes of a fresh and shiny look. The glowing sheen on my wavy tresses made me smile in the mirror. I whipped my hair from left to right, making sure it was ready for all the dance moves. By the end of the performance two hours later, my hair had dried up like old grits in a southern grandmama's pot. Thankfully, the incredibly shrinking bush on my head did not prevent all the compliments from the neighborhood families. In the end, I was just happy with all the attention. I enjoyed having an occasion to shine.

I never believed I was ordinary. I don't think anyone is. Not really. My family made it seem like the people who founded Liberty Hill were ordinary. Maybe they were. But what those freed black men did, in 1871, was extraordinary. I marveled that the existence of our community was seen any other way. There weren't many extraordinary moments on Liberty Hill when I was a child. There were proud moments, tragic moments, even funny moments, but nothing extraordinary. Extraordinary meant different, and the residents of Liberty Hill did not like different. They did not like change. I wondered if this was why our boundaries were treasured and not explored.

I could see just beyond the stoplight and the railroad tracks every day. My Grandparents' house sat on the west end of Liberty Hill at the corner of Montague and Mixson Ave. Mama's house was on the east end facing the tracks. The thunderous roar of freight trains shook the house daily. I was accustomed to the little quakes so much, I rarely felt them. I often ran to the back porch or to the living room window to watch the big locomotives speed by.

Where are they going? I wondered.

I saw myself jumping on one of the moving boxcars and riding to the next destination. Fantasies of arriving in a new place with exciting adventures flooded my mind. I did not speak of these endless possibilities. I innately pursued it. The question repeated like a melodious verse. *What is life like beyond The Hill?* Finding the answer was a journey riddled with roadblocks and misdirection. But, the pursuit continued, despite it all.

Meet Mama

Sandra Smalls Porterfield was first and foremost, Sandra Smalls.

Mama was Sam and Ruth Smalls' only child after the death of their first little girl. They still had pictures of Gwendolyn before she died. I would sit on my grandparents' floor and stare at the old photos of their beautiful little girl. She was born with hydrocephalus; a massive amount of fluid on her brain which led to the common name, "water head baby." The effects were visible in the pictures. Her shiny, black hair covered a substantially larger head that affected her balance and limited her mobility. My favorite picture was one of her sitting on the same floor where I sat, looking into her eyes. It was easy to see past her condition because the joy shined brightly from the sweet face staring back at me. Most babies born with this disease were not expected to live past a year, but Gwendolyn defied all the odds. She lived to be seven years old. Though I never met her, I admired her. She proved everyone wrong by living beyond expectations. Still, her death had to be a blow for her parents. Grandmama talked with me about Gwendolyn. She talked about her strength and sweetness. Granddaddy never spoke about her. His focus was firmly on the daughter who remained.

The very core of Mama's identity was being "Sammy's daughter." My grandparents raised her with as many privileges as they could afford. Though this was not much for a black family on Liberty Hill during the 1950s and 1960s, it was more than enough for the Smalls family to be proud of. If Sandra wanted something, she told her father. He made sure she got it. This did not change when she married or when she became a mother. Mama married a U.S. Air Force soldier when she was 19. They had one child; my big brother, Cole, and divorced a couple of years later. When Mama could not be a parent, she took my brother to Sam and Ruth and they were his parents. Her second marriage, to a Marine, only lasted a year which was pervaded by physical abuse and a miscarriage. After the divorce, Sammy bought his daughter a house not far from his. It is the house where I grew up across from the railroad tracks. She lived in that house through her third marriage to my father.

Hosey Porterfield was a decorated Naval officer. Sandra worked as a waitress for Amtrak. Her job was convenient since the train station was on Liberty Hill. On Thursday nights, Daddy and I would drive her across Montague to the south side of Gaynor Street to drop her off. Mama seemed so glamorous to me, as she boarded the passenger car in her navy-blue pants suit with the large red bow tied around her collar. She glowed under the lights of the shelter. Daddy and I stood on the platform listening to the conductor say: "All aboard!" Occasionally, Daddy held my hand or picked me up to console me as we watched the train leave the station.

"You see her?" He'd say, pointing at the Amtrak car. Mama stood at the window for as long as she could, waving goodbye. She always returned on Sunday.

While Mama would be gone for a weekend, Daddy shipped out on Naval assignments for months. I enjoyed spending time with him when he was home. He was also a skilled wood and leather craftsman. When I was five, my favorite accessory was a belt Daddy made for me. I watched him at our kitchen table as he engraved my first name in 2D letters into the grain with tools from his hand. He finished it off with a beautiful flower vine detail around the length of the belt. The full-grain leather was a dark golden brown whose tree bark scent I could smell from my little waist as I pulled it through every pant loop.

I was still in kindergarten during Daddy's last memorable year in the house. It was a rollercoaster of family drama. Mama and Daddy did not physically fight or argue very much last year.

Conversations in our house were minimal since I told Mama that I saw Daddy kissing Rose while I was playing on my swing set.

Rose was Mama's best friend. She lived in a yellow house, two doors down the street. I spent many days at her house, eating supper and playing with her kids. It was fun and I looked forward to going over there most of the time. She and Mama shared meals, shopping trips, and child-rearing tips.

Once, after getting caught playing with Rose's gas stove, Mama and Rose decided to teach me a lesson about the danger of playing with fire. Mama sat quietly at the kitchen table, as Rose explained to me why I wasn't old enough to touch the stove. Occasionally, Mama slipped in her points, agreeing with everything Rose said. Rose did not yell or even raise her voice as she told me she was going to show me why the stove was so dangerous. Mama did not move from the table as Rose stood and walked towards me. She took my hand, led me to the stove, and turned it on. I heard the ticking of the pilot light as she held my hand and took a match. She lit the match with the burner. Then, she took my pointer and middle fingers. With the lit match, she circled my fingers and formed figure eights between them as the flame touched my fingers with every imaginary stroke.

I didn't make a sound as tears trailed down my little cheeks. I cried from the pain the fire caused on my fingers. I burned with anger and disgust as I watched my Mama sit at the kitchen table with her legs crossed and a cigarette in her hand, lit by the same match used just moments before.

Maybe I was still angry when I saw Daddy kissing Rose on her back porch. I was on my swing set in our backyard. Southern neighborhoods of the early '80s were houses with yards that were open and spacious. Liberty Hill was no different. I could see clear across our next-door neighbor's yard, right onto Rose's back porch. It was a clear sunny afternoon as I swung carelessly with my braided ponytails flying in the breeze. When I noticed them on the back porch, I didn't think anything was out of the ordinary. Yet, as the

7

kiss grew longer, my mind was curious with questions. I jumped off the swing, mid-air, and ran into the house for answers from Mama.

"Mama, why is Daddy kissing Rose like that."

She scrunched her face in confusion, "What?"

"I just saw Daddy kissing Rose on her back porch."

"Are you sure," she asked? Her brow was still low. Her face was tight.

"Yes, Ma'am. I saw them. They were kissing like they do on TV."

She was quiet for a bit. Then she lifted her brow and nodded.

"OK, baby," she smiled and said. "Don't worry about it. I'll ask your Daddy for you."

I was confused until I realized what was happening. I wasn't valedictorian at my Christian kindergarten for nothing. They taught us all 10 commandments, and I remembered every one of them.

"Was Daddy committing adultery," I asked?

"I said, don't worry about it, baby. I'll handle yo' Daddy."

I didn't need a yes or no. She answered that question and a few others I didn't get a chance to ask. Yes, Daddy was committing adultery. Yes, he was going straight to Hell for it. And Mama was going to be the one to send him. My only question was, *when?* I got my answer on a bright Sunday morning.

Our family was preparing for church, but Mama was running unusually late. She was still walking around the house in her white waffle robe when she finally announced,

"I'm not going to church today."

My father didn't question her.

He simply said, "OK," then picked up his keys at the door and called for me to join him.

"Oh, she's coming," Mama said.

As she headed towards the door, I ran out of my room behind her. Church was always a fun event for me. I bolted off with excitement when the back door opened. Suddenly, I felt the back of my dress being tugged so hard, I nearly fell backward. Instead of jumping into Daddy's pale blue Buick, I was staring at the red crest on Mama's robe pocket. She stood with her feet planted firmly in front of me as she yelled out the door.

"Wait a minute!"

My father had cranked up the car only seconds before he stepped out to see what Mama wanted. I suppose he always knew. Inside Mama's little frame was a power-packed woman. That Sunday, he found out just how much she was packing.

Mama slid the .45 revolver out of her red-crested pocket. She pulled the trigger so calmly, it seemed effortless. Her hands did not shake one bit when the windshield cracked from the piercing bullets. Daddy didn't shake either when he darted into that Buick and floored it, in reverse, out of the front yard.

Then, just as calmly as she had pulled it out, Mama placed the gun back into her pocket, locked the door, and led me into the house. I never saw the police come for Mama. Daddy never came back into the house again. Soon after, they filed for divorce. Years later, my father married Rose.

I did not ask questions about that Sunday. I didn't have any. Maybe most five-year-olds would not comprehend it, but I knew exactly what happened. I always understood they had nothing to do with me. So, I never felt a need to question anyone about it. Hosey was still my father but his role in my life was done. Mama's role, however, had only just begun. I would have many questions about that.

Control

I waited for Mama at my grandparents' house on the day her marriage was officially over. Mama walked through the door with a big smile on her face. She made the process seem so simple.

"How was it?" I asked.

"It was fine," she replied with a smile. "I am officially divorced." My little mind needed details.

"So, what did you do? Did you and Daddy have to say different vows or say the opposite of what you said at the wedding?"

"Nooo," Mama replied, laughing. "You just sign some papers. That's it."

She placed her purse on the dining room table and went back into the kitchen to see what her mother cooked for dinner.

For a while, after Daddy left, on Saturday mornings Mama and I went to what looked like someone's house from the outside. Inside was not welcoming at all. It was too quiet. The crème painted walls were formal and stiff. Nothing about it felt like anyone's home. A white lady greeted us when we arrived. She spoke with me, alone, for a little while during our first visit. She asked how I felt about Mama and Daddy breaking up. I told her the truth. I really didn't care, and I'd rather be watching cartoons.

Mama made me go to the follow-up appointments just in case the lady wanted to talk to me again. I spent every hour sitting in the front room of the house. The shelves were full of books and magazines that were of no interest to a six-year-old. Meanwhile, Mama would be in the other room talking with the lady. Sometimes, I tip-toed to the closed door and tried to listen to their conversation. I heard their voices, but I could not make out the words. The hour felt like forever until the door opened. Mama never gave many

10

details about what they talked about in the room. She never gave details about much of anything.

A year passed before Mama brought Willie home. I didn't like him when we first met. I was seven years old and had grown accustomed to life with just Mama and me. Also, I could not believe his real name was Willie Williams. It sounded like he should be singing on stage somewhere. The first night, he tried to talk to me in the den while I sat in the little leather chair my father made just for me. I looked at the tall, dark-skinned man and refused to grace him with full conversation. Instead, I shot piercing looks of disapproval which made him retreat for the night. But Willie did not give up. He gave me time. Each day he came to the house, he acknowledged me and respected my lack of trust. This, in turn, made me respect him. He slowly won me over with his gentle spirit. It gave our relationship a strong foundation built on his patience and kind heart. Growing up, I told him everything, from my goals and dreams to problems with boys. He genuinely listened.

Our greatest conversations were during long walks through the back streets of Liberty Hill. He told me stories about different people in the neighborhood. We talked about history and family. The more time I spent with Willie, the more I wanted to know about him. I probed for details about his life. *Who was 'B' in the heart tattoo on his arm? Why did he leave school in the seventh grade? Was he happy with his life now?*

"You sho' ask a lot of questions," he would say. But he always told me what I wanted to know. He was not ashamed of his past or his mistakes. He tried to learn from them.

When I was eight years old, I asked Willie if I could call him "Daddy." We were at my Grandparents' house. I sat on the small sofa in the den, watching Willie fix a broken radio for me. The afternoon sunlight shone on him through the window behind me and he looked like the father I wanted. So, I asked.

"Willie," I said nervously. "Can I call you Daddy?"

"You can call me whatever you wanna call me," he answered, not looking up from the radio.

I tried it for a few days but soon settled on calling him by his first name. The title 'Daddy' was uncomfortable to me for a lot of reasons. One, I don't think Willie was comfortable with it either. His mouth tensed up around the edges when I said the word. Also, I never let go of Hosey as my Daddy.

Mama loved me because I was her daughter, but she hated the part of me that was my father's. Hardly a day went by without her attacking any part of me that reminded her of Daddy. Her nose flared when anyone told her I looked like him. She often said I had a big head just like his. If I broke a glass or trinket, it was more than a mistake. The clumsiness could have only come from my father.

"Just like yo' stupid ass Daddy," she screamed every time I made her angry.

What made her happy was conjuring up ways to get back at my father. I was a very useful tool for her revenge. Her ideas seemed petty at first. In fifth grade, I realized how creative and well-planned they were.

I had not seen Daddy in three years. He called, unexpectedly, asking to spend some time together. Mama allowed him to come get me on a Teacher Workday. I was excited for the rest of the week. Willie was happy for me. He told me to enjoy this time with my Daddy. Mama had other advice. She said to make him buy me the most expensive thing I wanted. When the day came, I asked Daddy to take me to the mall. He bought me the British Knight sneakers I wanted from the moment they were released in 1987. I was happy to have them, but I wondered if he knew what Mama told me to do. Afterward, he took me to Chi Chi's Mexican Restaurant for lunch. We talked about school and church. His smile was wide all afternoon. I smiled too. It was a beautiful day together.

The next morning, I was preparing for school. I fixed my lunch, as usual, and was eating breakfast. Mama came into the kitchen.

"You almost ready for school?" She asked.

"Yes, ma'am," I said.

She walked around to the side of the table where I was sitting.

"Come here, Quala."

I knelt with her on the floor. I thought we were going to pray. We were kneeling next to the huge pink cotton roll wrapped in a strange paper with Pink Panther on the front. Mama turned me with the side of my face next to the roll.

"Ok, close your eyes," she said.

She took my face and pushed it against the big roll. Slowly, she began to rub my face, back and forth, on the roll. My face began to itch and sting.

"Mama, what are you doing?"

"Shut up, Quala," she snapped. "Just do what I tell you to do. Keep yo' eyes closed."

She continued to rub my face against what I remembered Willie bought to insulate the house. After a few more seconds, we got up. She took a good look at my face.

"Good. Now don't tell anyone what happened to your face. You hear me?"

"Ok," I said, reaching up to touch it.

"No!" Mama slapped my hand down. "Don't scratch it. You can't scratch it. You'll make it worse. Just leave it alone."

I wasn't in school long before a teacher noticed the side of my face. She immediately sent me to the nurse.

"What happened to your face, Ruthenna?" she asked as she examined the strange appearance. The nurse tilted my head from side to side.

"I don't know." I was honest. I had no idea why Mama rubbed my face against home insulation. She told me not to say anything, so I didn't.

"Well, it looks like some type of allergic reaction. I'll call your mother. She'll have to take you to the emergency room."

13

Mama arrived at the school and had a short discussion with the nurse. She asked Mama if I had eaten anything different in the past twenty-four hours.

"No," she answered. "Not that I know of."

"Well, has she been around any animals or anyone different or new?"

Bingo! This was what Mama was waiting to hear. The day before, I had my first court-appointed visit with my father since the divorce.

"The only different person she's been around is her father. Yesterday was the first time she saw him in a long time."

"Hmm," the nurse said as she wrote her notes. "You definitely want to take her to the emergency room."

Mama thanked the nurse and took me straight to the Naval Hospital.

The conversation was similar with the doctors and nurses there. They asked me what I ate with my father and if he touched my face. I had not eaten anything out of the ordinary. Daddy hugged me but that was all. Then the doctors gave Mama something to use for my face. They also advised her to keep me away from anything new for the time being. To Mama, this included my father. But Daddy did not give up.

A few months later, a court order allowed me to go to his house every other Saturday and stay until Sunday. The law overruled Mama's authority and revenge. I looked forward to weekends with Daddy. We went to the Naval Base on Saturday mornings. He always fixed a grilled cheese sandwich for me in the afternoons. I treasured them almost as much as the leather belt with my name on it. On Sunday, he took me to his church before dropping me off at home by two o'clock. I got to know my father for six months. Then, one weekend, Mama said he was not coming. When I asked why, her answer was simple.

"Yo' Daddy don't give a damn about you," she exclaimed.

14

I turned eleven without hearing from Daddy. Mama's explanation started to make sense. If he doesn't want to see me, he must not care. It was genuine childhood logic. Eventually, I lost the leather belt. I latched on to Willie's love instead.

Willie was not my stepfather in the traditional sense. He and Mama never married. Their on-again, off-again relationship periodically added to the drama of our home for nine years. Anytime Mama wanted to feel more control over Willie, she simply threw him out of the house. If he didn't bring her enough money, she threw him out of the house. If he drank too much, she threw him out of the house. If she just felt like asserting her space and independence, she threw him out of the house. Nevertheless, Willie always came back. This was a mystery to me. He was a decent-looking man who never married or had any children. He was a hard worker. Flawed like everyone else, but he was a good man. He could undoubtedly have someone who treated him better than Mama, but Willie wanted Sandra Smalls.

I didn't learn much about love while living with those two. Willie was in love with Mama. I was not so sure those feelings were reciprocated. She cared about him, but Mama made it quite clear she would not marry him. A big reason was his drinking problem. Willie had a weakness for beer and lots of it. He did not drink much during the week, but Friday nights were different. Willie loved to go to Ed Lee's club. If he was not there, he was at "The Hole" which was just a tree stump in a vacant, grass-covered lot on Liberty Hill, on the southwest end near the railroad tracks. It was where men gambled their checks away, playing dice or Tonk.

I always got nervous as the hours passed and he was not home. At some point, there would be a loud banging on the back door. In my room, I would hear Mama walk down the hall to the kitchen.

"Who is it?" she'd yell.

She always knew who it was. If the door never opened, I knew Willie was drunk. She didn't have to open the door to know he had been drinking. His voice went up an octave when he drank too much. Sometimes, he came to my window and asked me to open the door. I just told him to go away. The phone would ring a few minutes later. He called from a nearby phone booth. I answered because Mama refused. He always said the same things.

"Put yo' Mama on the phone," or "Come open the door."
The phone calls were pointless. If Willie was drunk, he probably would not get in the house again until Sunday.

Mama and Willie did not physically fight often. I never saw him lay a hand on her. I cannot say the same about the alternative. Mama was vicious. She used different weapons including her mouth. The names she spewed at him were cruel like 'dumb-ass drunk' or 'illiterate motha-fucka.' She sliced his arm with a kitchen knife. Bottles, pots, and pans were hurled at his head. Willie never fought back, though he firmly held her at bay when necessary. One of their fights landed him in jail. Mama accepted his collect calls while he was there. It was weird to hear their conversations. They talked as if their fight was not the reason he was in jail. He asked how we were doing. She told him about what was happening on Liberty Hill. He was released after a short period, and life went back to normal like nothing ever happened.

Mama kept Willie around, partly, because of his close relationship with me. But she was not pleased with it. I talked with him more than her and she noticed. She never went on walks with us. She didn't laugh at our jokes. Our relationship was one of the few things in her house she could not control. This was not for lack of trying. Throughout my elementary school years, she interrupted conversations for no apparent reason. She did not invite him to my award ceremonies or speaking competitions. She never allowed me to put up pictures of Willie and me. Willie was not bothered by her efforts nearly as much as I was. When I complained to him about what she did, he calmly talked to me until I let it go. He understood what I was still learning about Mama. Sandra Smalls Porterfield was the queen, and her authority was not to be questioned.

Sibling Rivalry

The one place Mama knew her authority was limited was my Grandparents' house. I was there every day. Mama was able to keep a certain amount of authority at my Grandparents' house when it came to me. Whenever she felt her power was threatened, she snatched me up and drove me home. Her son, however, was a different story.

After Mama's first marriage was over, she decided motherhood was over too. So, my brother's weekend sleepovers at our grandparents' turned into a lifetime living arrangement. Cole was eight years older than me. Grandmama and Granddaddy raised him. Their house was his home. There were times he spent the night at our house, but those nights were rare. He loved his house, and he loved his parents. Cole loved Mama too, but not in the same way I loved our mother. I noticed the difference during an extended stay with Grandmama.

More than a week had passed since I saw Mama. I always liked being at my Grandparents' house, but this time was different. It felt a little too long. I asked my grandmother when Mama was coming to take me home.

"It's go'n be a little while, baby," she answered.

"Well, why can't I just stay with Willie?" I continued to probe.

"It ain't right for an eight-year-old girl to stay with a man in a house."

Her answer made me mad.

"But he's my stepdaddy!" I snapped.

"Hey," she snapped back! "Watch yo' mouth. They ain't married. And he ain't your…"

Grandmama stopped when she saw my eyes well up with tears. Finally, she sat me down and told me the truth.

"Quala, your Mama had a nervous breakdown."

"What's a nervous breakdown?" I asked.

"It means she got a little sick in her head and we had to send her to the hospital to rest so she can get better."

I heard everyone saying "nervous breakdown" around the house. I thought it was the same as Grandmama's hand-shaking. She said they shook because she was nervous or because her nerves were bad. Hearing "sick in the head" made Mama sound crazy. Grandmama said not to worry. We were going to see her on Saturday or Sunday. I was concerned but my brother seemed unfazed. He did not ask any questions.

The weekend came and I piled into the car with Willie, my grandparents, and Cole. We drove two hours to Columbia, South Carolina to see Mama. We passed a sign with the words "Department of Mental Health," but it did not look like what I expected. There were beautiful, lush, green lawns on either side of the road. We parked and walked towards a large building that looked like it was a part of a summer camp. There were high ceilings with wood beams. Though it was not the crazy house I pictured from television shows, I still wondered if Mama would come out to us in a straitjacket. Much to my relief, she walked through two glass doors with her arms free. Cole smiled. His eyes did not light up, like mine, when she came out.

We went outside and sat on a long bench. Just beyond the lawn was a forest of more trees reaching to the blue sky. The day was beautiful. No one talked about why we were there. We talked about what was happening on Liberty Hill. A bird mistook Willie's outstretched arm for a toilet which made us laugh. It was one of the few times Cole seemed connected. He was quiet most of the afternoon, focused on the trees or the grass in the distance. Cole was present but somehow, not with us.

I understood Cole was my brother, even though we lived in separate homes. This was not foreign to me. I had three more sisters

19

and another brother who also lived in a different house. They were my father's kids from his marriage before Mama. No one told me they were stepsiblings. When someone asked how many siblings I had, my answer was always three sisters and two brothers.

Mama kept an old Polaroid of all five of my siblings when they were little. The picture was taken only months before I was born. They were standing in Granddaddy's yard on a hot spring day. My oldest sister, Tee, towered over everyone foreshadowing how mature she would become. Shawn was closest to Cole in age. They stood next to each other cheesing to the camera. My other brother, Marcus, stood in front with a sweet and innocent smile. People often said he had the strongest resemblance to my father. Next to him was Tasha. She was the youngest at four years old. All the kids' eyes had a playful joy in that picture. It was like getting a glimpse of how my sisters' and brothers' bond was formed.

I spent more time with Cole than my other siblings because we shared the same mother. We saw each other every day when I went to my Grandparent's house. Days began at Grandmama's breakfast table, wolfing down her grits before heading out for school. In the afternoons, we were at the dinner table enjoying her rice and cornbread. This was after arguing over the Bible verse Grandmama required us to say after grace and before taking a bite. We were not allowed to say the same verse as anyone else. Each day, my brother and I raced to say the shortest verse in the Bible, "Jesus wept." After a few days, Grandmama would make us say something different. By the next week, the race would be on again.

My favorite word to use about my brother was "aggravating." Grandmama said it when I tattled on Cole. I did not know exactly what it meant, but I knew my brother was doing it. Anytime he hit me, took something from me, or would not play with me, I yelled in frustration.

"Stop aggravating me!"

"You don't even know what that means!" He usually responded.

This led to a shouting match that Cole would end by locking me out of his room. The next day, I was back at the house and the whole thing started all over.

The lock on Cole's door was one of many things he received from our Grandparents. He became their second child and only son. My Grandparents were raising Cole the same way they raised my mother. If he wanted something, Grandmama and Granddaddy got it for him, and it led to two major problems. The first was a sense of entitlement my brother developed. It eventually backfired on him. The second problem was a unique and complicated relationship between him and Mama. They did not share a parent and child bond. It was more like a strange sibling rivalry that often erupted in all-out war.

One afternoon when I was eleven years old, I heard the battle lines being drawn while playing in my Grandparents' den. Cole wanted to go somewhere, and he asked Grandmama for permission. It was a simple request made in Mama's presence. Suddenly, my brother was yelling.

"You can't tell me what to do!"

What should have been a quick exchange turned into a heated power struggle. Mama and Cole's shouting was so loud it traveled from the kitchen, down the hall, and into the den where I was playing. By age eleven, I had seen enough family drama to know when the real action was coming.

The bangs and thuds began to drown out the song playing on my little boom box. I turned the radio off, sat on the sofa, and did not move. I wasn't afraid, but very curious. My first thoughts were anger and concern.

"Grandmama better not be in the middle of their fight," I said to myself.

But my anger quickly subsided when I heard her yelling.

"Y'all need to stop all this!"

At sixty-nine years of age, my grandmother had no intention of getting in the middle of Mama and Cole's tussle. She still sat at the kitchen table while the two of them fought it out. I sat in the den and waited for their show to get in front of the door where I could see it.

"Get off me," Cole yelled.

The fight was making its way down the hall. By the time they were in my view, the two were so tangled in each other, I could not tell who had who. Finally, someone let go. Cole stormed past the den to his room. Mama tried to follow him, but he had already locked the door.

"Open this damn door," Mama yelled, as she tried to break into Cole's room.

"I paid for that damn door," Grandmama yelled back. "Y'all better not break a damn thing in my house."

Mama let go of the knob and thought for a few seconds.

"Ok," she said. "Alright, no problem."

She charged down the hall, through the kitchen, and out the back door.

It took a minute, but suddenly, her drastic logic was clear. We all darted outside at the sound of shattering glass. Grandmama, Cole, and I stood in shock as we watched Mama smash all the windows in Cole's new 1987 Chevrolet Caprice.

"Now," she said out of breath. "Fuck you and yo' car." She marched back into the house.

"Shit," Grandmama murmured. "I paid for the car, too."

This was the third car my grandparents bought for my brother. He wrecked the first two. I waited for Cole to say something: to yell, to cry, to go after Mama. He did not do a thing in front of me. He just started walking. Grandmama tried to console him as he headed out of the yard. If Sandra was Sammy's baby, Cole was definitely Ruth's

"It's alright, Cole. Just go rest your nerves. I'll talk to your Mama." Cole, silently, walked out of the yard.

Grandmama went back into the house. She was still trying to talk some sense into Mama when Granddaddy came home. We explained the whole thing to him, but there was no getting through to Mama.

"So, where Cole at now," Granddaddy asked?

Grandmama answered, "I don't know."

"Oh, Lord." Granddaddy said, shaking his head.

Mama and I went home a little later. When we got out of the car, she was still pleased with what she had done. The house was unusually chilly when we walked in.

"Mama, it's kinda cold in here."

"Yeah, I'll turn the heat on."

She was placing a dish in the kitchen sink when I heard her exclaim, "This mutha…Oh, I know mutha fuckin' well…"

She started marching again. I followed her out the door and around the house. Broken glass was on the ground, in front of every other window. Though the Protecto-Guard prevented any major damage, the point was clearly made. Cole won.

There were never any apologies from either side. All the windows on the house and Cole's car were eventually repaired. This battle was over, but there were always more. Each one followed the same pattern ending with damage, repair, and no apologies. I hated the war between Mama and Cole. I wanted them to get along like a normal mother and son, but they were not normal. I decided to just be happy when they weren't fighting, even in times of tragedy. It provided a little proof of love between them.

Tragedy struck hard a few months after the car battle. Grandmama smoked cigarettes for decades and the habit caught up to her. She had lung cancer. I heard her complain about arthritis before she got noticeably sick. Her hands still shook from old nerve problems and the pain she was in was excruciating. Grandmama would lie in bed for hours, trying to sleep away the pain. When she couldn't sleep, it was almost unbearable to watch. But I did watch, once.

I was in the kitchen adjacent to her bedroom. Her moans of anguish were soft but audible. The door was open, but I did not go in. The room was dark, and it seemed even the slightest sound or movement would cause more pain. So, I stood and watched my Grandmama. Her eyes were closed tightly as her wrinkled hands squeezed the pillow next to her.

"Have mercy, Lord," she prayed. "Please Jesus. Have mercy." My grandmother's prayers were infamous. We often held family prayer meetings at her house. There were times when she woke everyone up at two or three o'clock in the morning to pray. All arguments and conflicts were put aside. If only for thirty minutes at 3 a.m., we had to be a united family. She always wanted that. She prayed for it.

But when Grandmama got sick, we had to pray for her. There were countless hours in the hospital. Many afternoons, Mama picked me up at the bus stop and took me straight to Baker Hospital to visit with Grandmama. On a Thursday in February, I got off the bus and Mama was waiting for me with one of her friends in the car. I got in the car and began chatting away about my sixth-grade math project I was working on and how I forgot French tutoring that afternoon.

"I need to talk to you, Quala," Mama said nervously. "You remember when I told you about the wheat and the tare and how God would separate them and…"

I vaguely remembered what she was talking about. Mama talked to me a lot about God and often tried to mimic Grandmama's prayer meetings at our house. She never really knew how to talk to me about anything. Most times, I just tuned her out or figured out the point she was trying to make, as I did in this instance. Her stalling had made the situation obvious.

"Grandmama died?" I interrupted her useless soliloquy. She turned and looked at me in the backseat, with a puzzled look on her face.

"Yes," she answered.

24

"Ok," I said. "You didn't have to go all around the mulberry bush."

I understood she was trying to soften the blow, but it was not necessary. I had prepared myself for the inevitable.

The funeral was on Valentine's Day in 1989. Mama let me pick a new dress and new shoes for the service. I was the only person in all white, sitting between my mother and stepfather. When the time came to view the remains, I walked up to the casket. I wasn't as afraid as I used to be at funerals. A year earlier, an aunt passed away and her wake gave me nightmares. I was so scared, I went to Grandmama and asked her to promise not to come in my dreams if she died.

"Girl," she chuckled, "I'll be too busy enjoying my rest to bother you. But if it makes you feel better, I promise. And I'll make sure no one else bothers you either."

Her assurance made me walk up to see the body with ease. I was comforted even more when I looked at the face and it looked nothing like my Grandmama.

I smiled through my tears as I exclaimed, "That's just the body!"

My brother did not take it as well. I watched him walk up and take the 14K charm gold necklace off his neck. He placed it in the casket, and as he turned to go back to his seat, I focused on his face. Cole was more than saddened with grief. He was devastated with guilt. The woman he considered as his Mama was gone. He couldn't change the past or return the bail money she sacrificed for his various offenses. He couldn't pay her back for dropping out of high school or say thank you for spending time with his baby boy Jamal and getting him birthday presents when Cole didn't bother. Time was up.

As a pallbearer, Cole sat in pews on the right side of the aisle across from the rest of the family. Suddenly, Mama got up and walked over everyone in her way to get to Cole. More curious than concerned, I followed her across the aisle. Cole's hands were gripping the back of his head and his face was filled with tears. His eyes were red and it seemed as if he could not breathe. Mama tried to hold him, but her presence was not enough. He wanted his *real* Mama. I hugged my brother tight. I realized this probably was the closest we would ever be to our mother.

Touched

The phone rang around seven o'clock in the evening. Daddy was on the other end. He called after hearing Grandmama was sick. Mama let me speak to him. We talked about school and the birthdays he missed. I told him how I still wore the leather belt he made for me. It was still my favorite thing to wear. He laughed at how a ten-year-old could still fit something from when she was five.

We talked about maybe spending some time together. I was excited at the idea. I did not care about the holidays that passed or the lack of birthday gifts. All I cared about was seeing my Daddy. I told him to hold on while I went to ask Mama. I saw red in her eyes as soon as I mentioned the idea. She did not answer. She just picked up the phone. I listened on the phone in the kitchen.

"Mutha fucka you must be out yo' mind," Mama yelled into the phone. "I gotta fight you to pay $300 a month and you talkin' bout seein' her."

Daddy tried but could not get a word in.

"You ain't seen her in God knows how long. Why you wanna see her now? Especially after what you did to her."

"What?! What did I do to her?" Daddy asked loudly.

"Oh, you wanna play stupid now. You know good and hell well what you did."

Daddy had no idea what she was talking about. But suddenly I did.

Almost a year before, Mama questioned me about what Daddy and I would do while she was away working for Amtrak. I repeatedly told her the typical stuff: Watching TV, reading, and going to church. I did not remember much about that time. She continued to drill me with questions about Daddy and me being together. Finally, she just asked if Daddy had ever touched me. I told her no, over and over. She kept at me and began to create the whole scenario for me. She made it sound like a story with the two characters but holes in the setting and dialogue. So I filled in the blanks. I wanted the story to be complete like the nighttime soaps I was allowed to watch, that a little girl should never see. She just smiled and told me how glad she was that I told her. I gave her the ace she needed and she was ready to play it.

I dropped the phone in the kitchen and ran to Mama's room.

"Stop, Mama! I have to tell you something."

"What? Hold on," she said, putting the receiver down. "What's wrong?"

"Daddy didn't touch me," I said through tears. "He never hurt me. I made it up."

She smirked.

"No, you didn't. But you know what you almost caused."

I was confused.

"You need to apologize to your father for what you did," she said as she picked up the phone. "Hosey, Quala has something to say to you."

I went back to the phone in the kitchen.

"Daddy, I'm so sorry." I was crying hysterically.

I told him about my false accusation of him molesting me. I apologized over and over for my horrible lie.

"Do you hate me?" I asked, still crying.

He paused for a second.

"No, let me talk to your mother."

I said okay and hung up. I went to my room feeling so awful and guilty. I was told so much about my father being a liar. I did not know if I should believe him when he said he did not hate me. It didn't matter because I hated myself. Why should Daddy pay for what someone else did?

***

A part of my grandmother's legacy was the gigantic role the church played in my upbringing. My weekends were consumed by church. I spent Saturdays in choir rehearsal and Sundays in service. If allowed, Sundays would be long days with Sunday School starting at ten o'clock in the morning. and worship service not ending until, sometimes, after four o'clock in the afternoon. This was a price for being a member of a Pentecostal Holiness church. My mother never paid that price. We left every Sunday at 2 p.m. sharp, regardless of what was going on in the service.

"Ain't nothing God can't get done by two o'clock." Mama would say, right before she got in her car to light up a cigarette and pull out the church parking lot towards home.

I loved being in church. I shined bright when I was there. Sunday School teachers always assigned me the longest Easter speech or the largest role in the Christmas play. During Sunday school review, I was always the first person to speak. I was also a soprano in the church choir.

The choir was led by a talented and charismatic young man. His Grandfather was the pastor of our church. The choir director was best known for his youth choir. We were a large group of kids, as young as six to as old as twenty. Invitations to sing came from all around the Tri-County area. We sang at church services and other choirs' programs, though nothing compared to our Anniversary Concert.

I was eight years old when I joined the choir. This was a family expectation. If your parents were members of our church, you were in the choir. It was not on Liberty Hill, but several residents were members. I knew all the 66 books of the Bible by the time I was five years old. I also learned how to shout and dance in the spirit which was called 'catching the Holy Ghost.' I suppose these were benefits of going to a Pentecostal Holiness church. I was trained by the best.

29

I watched the fancy footwork of fire-baptized believers all the time. They would dance up and down the aisles, in the pews, and on the choir stand. I listened to their testimonies which were little monologues about how good God was to them. They usually began with a song and a generic opening line.

"I wanna thank the Lord for wakin' me up this moanin' and startin' me on my way."

Then they went on about some sickness, usually arthritis in any limb or joint where it was possible to have pain. This inevitably led to some sort of prayer request and ended with a loud and affirming, "Amen," from the congregation.

Many choir members went to other churches. The choir director's talent and ability to nurture vocal talent in children was known around Charleston. Parents sent their children from everywhere in the city to be a part of his kids' choir. He knew how to train the youngest voices into singing machines. His training tactics during choir practice ranged from a little unorthodox to very extreme. Most parents blindly saw his tactics as a passion for music or a desire to see their children be the best singers. There were only a few insightful nay-sayers who pulled their sons and daughters after being informed of what would happen on Saturdays.

The understanding amongst the kids was what happened in rehearsal, stayed in rehearsal. A lot always happened on Saturdays. Rehearsals were like tent revivals with prayer, scripture readings, shouting, and dancing. The choir director was the preacher with his mini-sermons before the musical selections. We usually reviewed four to five songs and learned a new one. Reviewing one song could take almost an hour. Learning new songs occasionally took an hour and a half. Some Saturdays, I didn't get home until after eight in the evening.

Rehearsals lasted four to six hours for several reasons. First, much of the shouting and dancing took place during this time. If one person caught the Holy Ghost, we all caught the Holy Ghost. Kids ran around the church or jumped for joy in the choir stand. Since our choir director never wanted to "quench the Spirit" he would let this go on until we gathered ourselves to move on to the next song.

Also, a great deal of time was spent perfecting the songs. If we did not get a line right or a note in just the right pitch, we would go over that part again and again until it was to our director's liking. He would do whatever he thought was necessary to get us there. This is where his training tactics were mostly used. We would repeat one line, ten times. If a specific section was causing the problem, that section paid dearly.

I was a nine-year-old soprano, on a hot Saturday afternoon, when we were having trouble with a difficult chorus of an old song. Our section was singled out to repeat it over and over. There were around twelve of us and our young, adolescent voices were straining to sing the melodies. After fifteen minutes, the choir director stepped out of the sanctuary and returned with several cups of water. His tight jaw and curled brow said the water was not to soothe our worn vocal cords. The choir stand was silent.

"Keep singing," he yelled at the sopranos!

We began the chorus again. I felt another little girl's arm shaking next to me. He set the cups on the banister in front of us where we stood. Then he stood, looking down on each young face, and listened. He reached back for a cup, as we sang our little hearts out. Slowly, he poured just enough water on the first girl's neck and shoulders. He moved to the next one. And the next one. Finally, he got to me. The water was cold, falling down my collar and drenching my sleeve. We kept singing as he moved through the section. Finally, we sang the notes to his expectations with our shirts soaked and our faces wet with tears.

The water incident was on a long list of punishments. The choir director pushed kids down into the pews or yanked them out of the choir stand by their arms. We were constantly yelled at, for not singing but for mouthing or lip-syncing instead. When he felt someone was mouthing the words, each kid had to sing the part individually. Upon finding the kid who was struggling with the part, they would either be sat down or sent home, usually in tears. If he saw tears, he lashed out.

"What are you crying for," he would yell. "Maybe, if you sang as much as you cried, we'd sound better."

This sometimes turned into a lecture or sermon from the director who was in his early twenties. It started as a lecture about kids not singing and ended as a sermon about why we should not listen to any music other than Gospel music. He would compare those of us that he felt had talent to those who he felt could not hold a note. He singled out the kids he felt were saved to the kids he said were, "On their way to Hell." He often based their eternal damnation on a poor attendance record to rehearsals or singing engagements. If you did not fully commit to the choir, clearly you were not fully committed to God.

Dedication was a key to getting on his good side. I was at every practice and scheduled event. I idolized the choir director. This was much to my stepfather's dismay as he never liked him. Willie thought I spent too much time with the director and the choir. My mother did not listen to his suspicions, and I did not care about his concerns. I wanted to sing. I wanted to lead songs. I wanted to be in the limelight. Maybe getting on the director's good side could lead to my extraordinary moment.

A few weeks later, I came home to my grandmother's to find the choir director sitting in the living room. I was surprised and excited.

"What are you doing here?" I exclaimed.

"Your grandmother and your mother wanted me to talk to you."

Grandmama was on the couch next to him, across from Mama. *This could only be good*, I thought. *The choir director came to our house, just to talk to me.*

32

"You know, Ruthenna," he began, "You're a very smart young lady. You do well in school and that's good. You can go far with that."

"Thank you." I was so excited.

"And you do very well in the choir too. You're one of the loudest sopranos we have and you sing right in tune."

Things started to make sense in my mind, so I just asked, "So, does this mean I can lead a song now? You're here to tell me I get to lead?"

The choir director looked at the matriarchs for help. Mama shook her head. Grandmama tilted her chin and glared at him. He finally answered.

"Um, no Ruthenna," he said. "You cannot lead."

My heart sank. "But I don't understand. You just said I could sing."

"Yes, but not well enough to lead a song. You're a really good soprano, but it takes a special voice to lead."

"Like one of your favorites," I snapped, fighting the tears.

"Quala," My grandmother yelled!

The choir director had clear favorites. They were soloists. They were on the choir's Officer Board staffed with a president, vice-president, secretary, and treasurer among other positions held by children and teenagers. Officers were nominated by other choir members but approved by the director. He spent more personal time with the favorites, at their homes as well as his. He worked with them more to train their voices. These children were special. Every child wanted to be special, including me.

"No, it's ok," he said to my grandmother. "Ruthenna, you are one of my favorites. I love you. You know that. You're smart and very intelligent. But you cannot lead."

He was telling the truth. I was one of his favorites. Grandmama welcomed him into her home often. I was second vice president which felt like a true accomplishment to me at ten years old. The position made me feel important and needed. But being one of his favorites included much, much more.

As an officer in the choir, we had frequent leadership meetings. They were very formal and business-like. We discussed event attire, regulations, and fundraisers among other issues. We felt like adults in these meetings, though none of us were over 18, except the choir director and he was only twenty-one. Our choir director led the meetings, along with whoever was the president at the time.

I looked forward to a particular officer's meeting on a cloudy February afternoon in 1988. Everyone was supposed to bring their thoughts on fundraising and other choir events. I wrote my ideas down with excitement and placed them in a folder. It went into my blue, vinyl shoulder bag that seemed perfect for a business meeting. The rain was pouring when Grandmama pulled into the empty church parking lot.

"Nobody's here yet," she questioned.

"Maybe, I'm the first one here," I said excitedly.

We waited a few minutes until we noticed the light inside on the second floor of the education wing.

"Well, they must be here," Grandmama concluded. "Go in and I'll wait here 'till I see you in the window. Just call me when you're ready for me to pick you up."

"Ok, Grandmama. Love you!" I gave her a kiss or some "suga" as she called it. "Happy Birthday!" I opened the car door and charged through the rain to the back door of the church.

I went inside and upstairs to one of the classrooms. The officers' meetings were always held in the largest classroom because there was room to have a large table. I didn't see a table when I walked in this time; only chairs and the choir director sitting in one at the front of the room. I paused. For the first time in my young life, I felt a strange uneasiness. The air in the room was very unusual. I said hello to the choir director and went over to the window. Grandmama was getting out of the car until she saw me waving from above. I barely saw her through the rain as she waved back and got back into the car. The headlights shined bright enough to show how hard it was pouring outside. As she backed up, the strange uneasiness grew into a small feeling of butterflies and suddenly I had a strong desire to run back downstairs and outside to stop her, so I could go home. But in those few seconds, she had pulled off.

"Who you waving to, Ruthenna?"

"My Grandmama," I said, still looking out the window. "Today's her birthday."

"Really? Be sure to tell her I said, 'Happy Birthday.'"

I turned to him and smiled. "I will."

The butterflies were dwindling a little. He smiled back and told me to come over and have a seat. The air in the room felt warm and thick. I trudged over to the opposite side where he was and sat in a row of chairs directly across from him.

"Where is everybody else," I asked?

"I guess they're all late." He shrugged.

"Everybody?"

"I guess. They'll probably be here later, but you're the first one here."

"Oh." I was proud to be the only one on time. I smiled at the thought of being acknowledged for it once the meeting started. He saw my smile.

"What all is in your blue bag? You always bring it to practice and meetings."

The room was still strange, but I was excited by his interest.

"Well, my Bible of course. But I have all my notes from the meetings in a notebook. I have all my ideas, too." This was the chance I was waiting for. I started to take papers out. "I've been meaning to bring them up…"

"That's good," he interrupted. "You can bring them up at the meeting. I'm sure we can use them."

I pushed the papers back inside, disappointed. *At least, I'll be able to talk about them later*, I thought. Maybe we could work on some vocals until then.

We sat in silence for a few minutes. The room was shrinking as time passed. It slowly smothered my security. I could still hear the downpour outside when I noticed his eyes closed.

"Uh oh, are you falling asleep," I asked loudly?

He slowly opened his eyes. "No, I'm just resting my eyes."

I had passed his grandfather in the office next door to the room, but no one else had arrived. It seemed like a while had passed. I was ready to go home, but I did not want to say anything. What if the others finally showed up? What if I missed the meeting? Or worse, what if he didn't like me anymore because I wanted to leave?

I sat silent, watching his eyes close again.

Finally, he opened his eyes and looked straight at me.

"Ruthenna, come give me a hug." He opened his long arms. He was so tall, that even while sitting, he seemed huge. Even larger to a small framed ten-year-old girl.

I didn't move for a few seconds. I felt the uneasiness again, but it was stronger. Then, I reminded myself that he was like another big brother. He was only a couple of years older than my brother, Cole. He had been in our home. Grandmama adored him and so did I. His arms were still open.

I got up and walked over to him, still seated in the chair. I put my arms around his neck. He wrapped his arms around my tiny waist and pulled me against him in the chair between his legs. He held me for several minutes. I was immediately paralyzed with fear. *This was not right, was it? This was definitely off.*

He began to stroke my back. I felt one of his hands go lower on my back, stopping just short of my bottom. I almost wished he went further because then it would have been clear this was wrong. It was confusing. He slowly brought the other hand down, careful not to pass the first hand. I felt parts of him swelling. I did not know what it was at first. Then I realized it was his private parts.

He began to shift my body, slowly from side to side. I was so scared. He did not say a word, but I felt his hot breath on my neck. He did the same motion with his own body, but harder with me. So many questions went through my head. *Did he do this with all of his favorites? Why did this feel funny?* There were rumors and headlines about him in the last year. *Had he really done this to the girl he allowed me and others to lie about to attorneys?* He held me tighter as he continued shifting and moving our bodies.

I thought about the night, about a year before, in the church van on the way home from practice. My brother drove while the choir director sat in the front passenger seat. The choir director asked if I had ever kissed anyone.

"Of course," I told him.

He explained that he meant people other than my family, like boys. I told him no. He said I needed to practice and that I should practice with someone who loved me, like him, because he would never hurt me. He put his mouth on mine. I was so horrified; I would not open my mouth. He stopped and told me to relax and open my mouth because it was natural. I thought about how Mama sat watching Rose so many years ago. Cole drove the church van in silence on this night. The next time I followed his instructions as he put his tongue in my mouth. He asked how it felt.

"Tingly, right?" It was not tingly, it was disgusting. And so was this rainy afternoon.

I did not want him to put his mouth on me again, so I decided to stop him before he did. I couldn't think of anything and was too scared to do something drastic. It had to be done right. Distraction was the only thing to make him stop. He was still moving and shifting my body on his. I began doing the alphabet in sign language. When I got to the letter P, I did not remember the sign. I said his name. He immediately stopped, as I snapped him back to the present. His arms and hands were still clasped around me.

"Do you know the sign for the letter P?" I asked. He brought both his arms around in front of him to form a P with his two hands. He smiled at his signing attempt. I smiled too, to stay calm. I was free. I backed off of him and went back to my seat.

"No one's coming," I said. "I might as well go home."

I went to the office and asked his Grandfather, my pastor, to use the phone.

"You were the only one that showed up?" he asked.

"Yes sir," I said.

"Hmm."

I called Grandmama and waited downstairs until she came for me.

I only told one person what happened. I shared every problem with my sister during sleepovers. She was a caring listener. No matter what she was doing, Tasha always made time for me when I asked. And she always made a point to say, "I love you." Her love made it easy to trust her with what happened. I made her promise not to tell anyone. She was very apprehensive about keeping the secret. She said she would not say anything unless it happened again. It did happen again, and again. I never told her.

Grandmama lived eighteen days short of her next birthday. Mama called the choir director to the house. She wanted him to be waiting for me when I got back from school that day. She thought he would bring me comfort. He smiled when he saw me. I cringed. The choir director sang and played at Grandmama's funeral. He was the first person to walk up during the viewing. I watched him stop and look at my grandmother's body. He did not deserve to look at her. He did not deserve to live. I wanted to take Grandmama out of that casket and shove him in.

Mama finally joined another church a year later. By the time we settled into our new church, I had completely blocked the choir director out of my mind. Blocking it gave me a sense of power over him. I did not want him or what he did to control the rest of my life. There's power in choices. So, I chose to erase him from my existence. I went to our new church with my mother and a strong skepticism of every person I met on Sunday mornings.

The Other Side of the Tracks

When Grandmama was alive, we went on road trips to family reunions every July. Her relatives were scattered across the Deep South. She, along with Granddaddy, Mama, Cole and I piled into Granddaddy's Cadillac with a cooler stocked full of bologna sandwiches and sodas. We crossed the railroad tracks by nine o'clock in the morning and drove for six to eight hours. I sat in the back seat gazing at the different buildings we passed along the highways. A large, green sign always approached by noon. *Welcome to Georgia!* Hours later, we may see a sign welcoming us to Alabama and Florida depending on which cousin we were going to visit. Each family pilgrimage gave me a glimpse into the way other people lived.

I had no idea life was different off Liberty Hill until Mama transferred me to Buist Academy. In the spring of 1985, Mama heard Charleston County planned to open a new school for smart kids. A closed-down school building in downtown Charleston would be renovated for the project. Meanwhile, Liberty Hill School sat vacant for years, next to Bonds Wilson High which the county was closing at the end of the semester. I attended Berry Elementary, a mile north of Montague, with the other neighborhood kids. A math and reading test was required to be accepted into the new magnet school. I took the test and passed. Buist Academy for the Gifted and Talented opened in August, with me as one of the first third graders. Now, two vacant school buildings sat in my neighborhood.

I saw the abandoned structures every day. A tall metal fence surrounded the front of the school grounds. On my walks home, I stopped at the fence and tried to see through the walls. I thought about Mama's fond memories of caring teachers. I imagined Willie as a little boy, sitting in classrooms learning basic math. I walked a few feet down to the center of the fence where there was a chain and padlock. The entrance doors were several yards back behind overgrown grass and brown weeds. Sometimes, the grass grew so tall you barely saw the boarded windows. Months later, I walked past and saw the yard was cleared. The large letters spelling "Liberty Hill School" were visible once again.

Buist was a forty-minute bus ride from Liberty Hill to downtown Charleston. Every morning, Mama drove me to Park Circle Community Center, just beyond the stoplight, to catch the school bus. I wondered about the homes we passed as we crossed the Mixson Avenue intersection to the other side of Montague. Most of the wood structures were the same size as the ones on Liberty Hill. The square-shaped lawns were neatly kept like ours, though some had picket fences instead of metal. Things were different as we got closer to the traffic circle. Houses were made of dark red brick here. Some were two-story homes. The front yards were larger rectangles landscaped with full flower beds and green shrubbery. I saw homes like these on television.

"Who lives here?" I asked Mama one morning while driving around the circle.

"White people," she answered.

We turned into the parking area in front of Felix Davis Community Center. This center was vastly different from the one on the Hill. Felix Davis was twice the size of Felix Pinckney. The building sat in the middle of a round piece of land the size of a football field. A shiny swing set was on a large playground with a colorful sliding board. Trees stood tall around the nearly three-mile circle. We parked across from the community center to wait for the bus.

I saw more white people when the school bus arrived in the mornings. Kids with ivory hues were in line with me to board. The lady behind the big steering wheel greeted us with pale skin and dark hair. I walked through the doors at Buist and was welcomed by a white principal. At Berry, Mr. Willis was a nice black man who walked the halls constantly. I looked at this new principal and wondered if she would be mean to me. Miss Murray introduced herself at an assembly and proved to be kind like Mr. Willis. I was not.

I hated Buist Academy. Most of the kids knew each other from their previous elementary schools which made me feel like an outsider. None of my friends transferred with me from Berry. Leaving them made me angry and scared. So, I rebelled. In my first year, I was a tempered-driven terror. I did everything I could think of to get out of that school. I hit other third graders, argued with my teacher, and caused so much trouble on the school bus, I was nearly banned from riding it. When nothing worked, I became destructive.

The computer lab was nothing like any class at Berry Elementary. Fluorescent lights gleamed on the workspaces in the middle of the room. Twenty-five new computers were stationed on tables along the perimeter of the walls. An apple with a single bite slowly appeared when we pressed the button on the large monitors. Little chairs with shiny metal legs sat in front of each device. Our class went to the lab for one hour per week to practice typing and play a few educational games.

Paws was my favorite speed typing program. I enjoyed seeing the little cat feet struggle to keep up with the letters I sent to the screen. The fast, rhythmic clicking of the keys was soothing to me. One afternoon, the sound drowned out my teacher when she announced we were going back to class. Students lined up at the door. I stayed at the computer.

"Ruthenna," Miss Fike said sternly. "It's time to go. Turn off the computer and get in line."

I was indignant. *How dare she interrupt my game?* I didn't move.

"Now, Ruthenna." She spoke louder.

I felt my face getting hot and my breaths got shorter. This teacher was taking away the one thing I enjoyed at this school. Finally, my rage exploded. I picked up the keyboard and slammed it into the table. Keys flew into the air and landed on the floor. The loud crack echoed across the room followed by the gasps of third graders.

"Go to Miss Murray's office immediately." Miss Fike ordered. This was it. The principal would expel me for sure. I walked into her office, hopeful. To my dismay, Miss Murray simply called Mama and sent me home for the day. My third grade attempts to get kicked out were futile. I was not going anywhere. Four years later, I was still at Buist.

I looked forward to summers as my escape until sixth grade. Family road trips stopped after we buried Grandmama in February. Traveling anywhere seemed hopeless. Then one month before the end of the school year, Mrs. Dodd, the French teacher, announced she was organizing a small trip to Quebec, Canada for students. I was ecstatic. Mama cautiously entertained the idea by going to an interest meeting for parents.

"I'm not promising anything." Mama reminded me before we got into the car.

I put on my seatbelt with a wide smile. Just getting information was enough for me to remain optimistic.

The meeting was at the Circular Congregational Church in downtown Charleston. We parked on the grounds which was a palatial version of St. Peter's AME on Saunders Avenue. Both churches were historic staples of their cities, but the Circular Church seemed preserved. A cemetery surrounded the house of worship, crowded with hundreds of century-old gravestones. The brown brick was faded in some places but still sturdy. A colossal arch entrance connected to a three-story, hexagon tower on the left and a circular dome on the right. I was mesmerized by the round sanctuary where we met the other families. Mrs. Dodd's voice echoed off the high ceilings, as she softly explained the details of the trip.

At $1500, I thought Mama would turn her head, but she sat stone-faced with the white parents. Somehow, she came up with the money. Two days after the last day of sixth grade, my flight landed in Montreal. A chartered bus took more than forty students and chaperones to Quebec City. Everything I saw and ate was different. The grass on the rolling hills was more vibrant than at home. Cafés with outdoor seating covered by umbrellas lined the streets near our hotel. Sandwiches were flaky and succulent. I sat in a jacuzzi and a sauna for the first time. All the fantasies while watching the freight trains barrel by my house, were real. I returned to Liberty Hill knowing there was a life across the tracks that I wanted to live.

Seventh grade began with a whirlwind. On September 21, 1989, I came home from school with homework assigned by our science teacher. I was livid. The weather reports were adamant all week. Charleston lay in the direct path of Hurricane Hugo. The storm would hit tonight.

"How are we supposed to do homework?" I said to myself when the lights went out.

Hugo furiously ripped through the coast into the mainland. The loud whistle of the wind woke me up. The windows rattled so hard, it sounded like they would shatter. Then, at midnight, everything stopped. Silence. Mama and Willie went out to survey the damage as the storm's eye passed. Voices shouted through the darkness.

"Y'all alright?" People yelled down Gaynor Avenue.

"Yeah," Mama answered. "How 'bout you?"

"We good, so far."

Suddenly, the wind began to blow again. Harder.

"Y'all betta get back inside now!" Willie exclaimed.

Sheets of rain poured down as everyone ran back into their homes. The hurricane barreled across the tri-county area for the rest of the night.

The day after the storm, Liberty Hill was in shambles. There was no electricity. Trees were down everywhere. Yards were flooded and homes were nearly destroyed. Somehow, that Friday morning was amazingly beautiful. It was a warm day and the sun shined bright in the clear, crisp, blue sky. While only a few shingles came off Mama's roof, my Grandparents' house took a major blow.

Cole was home during the storm with his girlfriend and her baby girl. When Mama, Willie, and I went to check on them, we arrived at a disaster. Fallen trees and debris completely blocked the driveway. Granddaddy's yard was covered by a sea of broken limbs still full of foliage. We parked at Mr. McCant's old filling station next door. Willie grabbed the saw out of the trunk of the car. He cut branches, one by one, clearing a small path through the yard to the back door. A strong scent of wet flower blooms permeated the house when we walked into the kitchen.

"Cole?" Willie called out.

"Yeah, we back here!" My brother responded.

We continued to the living room where we were greeted by the source of the smell. A huge tree stood upside down through the ceiling onto the green carpet. Hurricane wind gusts sliced part of the Magnolia tree in the front yard and sent the crown crashing through the roof. Little rows of light peaked through the rafters holding up the trunk. Shards of glass from the blown-out window were on Grandmama's old sofa. Thankfully, everyone was in the back of the house, away from the danger during the storm.

Like all the black neighborhoods in Charleston, Liberty Hill was one of the last to have its electricity restored. This was painfully clear when I spoke with my white friend from school. Renee lived twelve miles north in Hanahan. The city was nicknamed 'Klanahan,' in part for the scarcity of black residents there. Two weeks after Hugo hit, I sat in my bedroom lit by candles and listened intently to Renee watching a new episode of *The Cosby Show* as it premiered on television Thursday night. Her laughter stung when it came loudly through the receiver. I rushed off the phone when the show was over.

"It's not fair," I told Mama when I got off.

"I know, baby." She said, shaking her head.

The lights were on in houses on the other side of the railroad tracks. Streets were brightly lit across Mixson Avenue. Liberty Hill residents sat in the dark for a month.

Despite the unfair system, the neighborhood stood with the pride of the people who built it. Neighbors threw cookouts for each other until the power came back. Adults worked together to clean up the wreckage from the storm and make sure elderly residents had everything they needed. Our lights finally flickered on a week before Halloween. There were two months left in 1989; still enough time for craziness before the start of a new decade.

Mama vs. Me

Bone cancer came for Granddaddy. He was in the hospital for a short while after repairing the damage from the storm. Agonizing pain shot through his legs so much, he could barely walk. Mama moved us into his house to help him recover. The doctors sent him home with needles and vials filled with codeine. Mama tried to teach me how to give him the shot. She said it was important for Cole and me to learn in case we were home alone with Granddaddy when he needed it. We sat at the kitchen table with everything laid out. She showed me how to get the medicine out of the vial and where to stick the needle. Cole did it once and then went back to his room.

"Ok. Now you try," she said, handing me a practice needle filled with water.

My little hands were shaking. All I had to do was slowly push the fluid out into a cup on the table.

"Come on, Quala." Mama said with frustration.

My hands shook as I pushed the water out and quickly put the needle on the table.

"I don't want to do this, Mama," I said in tears.

"You just did."

"What if I put the needle in the wrong place on Granddaddy? What if I give him too much? I can't do it. Please," I begged.

"Ok. Fine," Mama replied, frustrated. "You don't have to do it."

I got up from the table, still crying, and retreated to my brother's room. I liked staying in Cole's room. It made us feel like real siblings. Staying at Granddaddy's also kept Mama distracted. Her focus on taking care of her daddy provided a temporary cease-fire between her and her children.

Battles between Mama and Cole subsided after Grandmama died. Sleepovers and daily visits ended. We went over a few times a week before Granddaddy fell ill. My brother was rarely home when we stopped by. They argued occasionally but it never escalated because they were not together long enough. I became Mama's sole target. I felt like my childhood was a constant war with her. Ironically, for me to win each battle, she had to be happy. If she was happy, she didn't yell at me. If she was happy, she didn't belittle me. If she was happy, she didn't hit me. Winning did not always feel like a victory. It just felt like survival.

Willie tried to protect me from Mama's spontaneous fury by occasionally taking me out of the house. On Christmas Day, he wanted me to spend some time with his family. I loved the Williams-Broughton clan. They were a loud, humorous bunch of folks who were all pretty much like Willie. The men were drinkers. The women were talkers (some were drinkers, too.) And no one was afraid to speak their mind. Family gatherings were filled with hysterical honesty and lots of love. I could not wait for my first Christmas with them.

Cole and I opened gifts early in the morning. Granddaddy was more mobile after a month of physical therapy. A walker helped him move to the dining room table for dinner. Willie came by during our feast and asked Mama if I could go with him to his sister's house afterward. She said it was fine. I never ate so fast. I grabbed my coat and pranced out the door behind him. The Williams-Broughton family gathered at the home of Willie's older sister, Liz. When we arrived, Christmas was in full swing. The house was filled with people. Large foil trays of sliced turkey, collard greens, sweet yams, and red rice sat on every table and countertop. Kids were running from room to room. The teenagers were watching BET music videos. Some of the adults played hosts in the kitchen as people walked through the door. Others were playing a rowdy game of Spades or just talking in the living room by the Christmas tree where presents were waiting to be revealed for the family's secret Santa. Since I was going to be a teenager in eight months, I decided to join the others on the den sofa to hopefully catch my favorite song on television. I was sitting for less than thirty minutes when Willie came over to me.

"I think you better call yo' Mama."

"Why?" I asked.

"Just to let her know you over here."

I still did not understand, but I went to the phone to dial the number. I barely heard her answer with all the excitement around me.

"Mama, we're at Liz's house." I tried to speak so she could hear. Laughter burst through the background, and she asked, "What's all that noise?"

"We're about to open presents," I exclaimed.

She paused and then angrily ordered, "Bring yo' ass home!"

I was shocked. "Huh?!"

"You heard what I said."

"But, why?" A lump formed in my throat as my eyes welled up.

"Cause I'm yo' Mama," she declared. "Put Willie on the phone." I put the phone down and told Willie what she had said. He shook his head and went to the phone. He tried to reason with her, but it was no use. Bitter frustration was written on his face as he hung up.

"Come on. I gotta take you back home." Willie said with his head down.

I was angry and devastated. Cold tears streamed down my face during the slow walk back to Granddaddy's house. Willie dropped me off without saying a word. I saw a smile on Mama's face as I walked past her to my brother's room. I cried on Tony's bed through Christmas night.

New Year's Day came, and Mama moved us back home. The second school semester began with the annual Science and Math Fairs. Every student picked a topic to research and experiment with.

I chose surveys and graphs for a math project because I figured it was the easiest thing to do. Ask a bunch of people about a subject and report my findings on a graph. Only one question interested me enough to search for an answer. Why were Liberty Hill School and Bonds Wilson High still closed?

The elementary school had been closed for decades, but Bonds Wilson was the pride of Liberty Hill. My family lit up when they talked about their days in high school. Residents used the empty student parking lot to teach their teenagers how to drive. Graduates, from the previous generation, still wore their letter jackets. All the neighbors thought of the school as their own. They spoke fondly of the unity Bonds Wilson High built among the residents of the neighborhood. They wanted to pass it down to their children.

Mama gladly took me to the old school properties to take pictures for the project. A dilapidated breezeway stretched from the rear entrance of Liberty Hill School to Bonds Wilson. The high school property began a little off The Hill's border. Its front and back gates were always open. People drove through to get to another side of North Charleston. I rode my bicycle in the school's abandoned parking lot often as a little girl.

I would park my bike at the front gate and walk towards the buildings. All the windows on Liberty Hill School were boarded but there were a few on Bonds Wilson that were not. Occasionally, when I was not spooked, I peeked through the glass of the front entrance doors. I could see the wide hallways and the tattered sign directing visitors to the office. If I felt really brave, I rode around the side of the high school property. The windows to the empty cafeteria were still open. As I stared in the windows, I imagined hundreds of students sitting at the tables eating hot lunches. I heard the loud chatter of teenage gossip. I turned around and saw the tall, rusted spotlights towering above the overgrown football field. I imagined the sound of the bell interrupting cafeteria conversations about the next game.

Around the corner from the cafeteria was a bright red, free-standing structure. Three or four steps led to the small entrance door. Inside was a mystery because there were no visible windows.

"What's this?" I asked Mama, walking towards the handrail.

"That's the old band room," she answered. "I never went in there. If you weren't a band member, you couldn't go in. I had to wait for my friends to come out."

Suddenly, I loved that building. It stood out from the rest of the school. The chipped red paint was like a stage curtain waiting to reveal something wonderful. A wide smile showed the gap in Mama's teeth as she told me about watching the band march from the band room to the field every Friday night.

Charleston County School Board sent shock waves around the city when they decided to close Bonds Wilson in 1985. The plan was to merge this neighborhood beacon with the predominately white North Charleston High (NCHS), located only a few miles away. Liberty Hill was crushed. Bonds Wilson's closure represented another iconic entity in the black community that was snatched by the powers of a white system. It was a hard blow to the pride of a neighborhood.

For my math project, I knocked on more than twenty doors to talk about the closed schools. Everyone agreed they should be reopened. Some offered suggestions such as using the structures for offices like how Buist was used before it was renovated into the magnet school. Others said the buildings could be converted to a trade school. There were many options but one consensus. None of this would ever happen. Residents saw the boarded windows every day and were despondent. I heard it in every dismal conversation and pointless complaint.

"Them white folks ain't go'n let us have nothing."

Pride in the past with no hope for the future equaled no progress. Claustrophobic anxiety made my shoulders tremble at their words. I did not want to be bound by the hopelessness resounding from my neighbors. The results of the survey were enough to get me a good grade and a resolve to get off The Hill. Eighth grade came and went. Finally, I left Buist with excitement about what was ahead.

I saw progress at North Charleston High. The school was rebuilt just before the merger with Bonds Wilson. The structure did not look like a typical high school. It looked like a new office building with a beautiful green lawn, welcoming students to the glass doors. The school motto was inscribed in the red stucco on the front of the building.

"EDUCATION IS A POSSESSION OF WHICH MAN CANNOT BE ROBBED."

The inscription intrigued me. I asked Mama what it meant.

"Can't nobody take away what you got up here," she said, tapping her pointer finger on the side of her forehead.

I thought about all the possibilities still hiding in my head from my fantasies watching the freight trains. My imagination would be free at North Charleston High. Every day would take me past the stoplight that stifled the dreams of a neighborhood. I had to go to this school.

Mama was not thrilled about me going to North Charleston High. Most of the eighth graders at Buist ended up at the new and growing Academic Magnet High School. I did not want four more years of the hell I went through at Buist. Mama was okay with me not going to the magnet school if there was a close educational equivalent. Her top choice was Ashley Hall, an all-girl private school in downtown Charleston. She scheduled a tour and time for me to take the entrance exam. The school grounds were beautiful, and the academics were stellar. But it did not have the spirit of NCHS. I found myself giving random answers on Ashley Hall's test. Lackluster results forced Mama to accept where I wanted to go. My freshman year at North Charleston High began in August.

I spent the summer before freshman year on the football field. Joining the Marching Cougar Band was a goal since the day I stood outside the bright, red structure with Mama. When Miss Simmons, the director, called to offer me a spot on the flag corps, I was ecstatic. School started after three grueling weeks of band camp. The first halftime show was two weeks later. After a few football games, more students recognized me in the halls. Everyone knew the skinny freshman girl who led the band on the field. Before long, the battles I fought at Buist Academy seemed like a distant memory. Unfortunately, the war at home still raged.

Many fights with Mama were ambush attacks. There were days she was loving and fun to be around. We watched movies together and went to gospel music concerts. Mama did not like to cook but she enjoyed making homemade apple turnovers. She hummed while pinching the edges before placing them in the oven. I loved our Saturday morning breakfasts at Waffle House. She always ordered her favorite pecan waffles. Sometimes, we went to Shoney's or Ruby Tuesday for dinner on a whim. She would be in the best of moods. Then, suddenly, she would explode.

One minute, I was walking in the new shoes she bought me. The next minute, my face was swollen because I wasn't walking in the heels right. Anything could set her off. A question might receive a slapping answer. What I chose to wear for the day led to tirades about how bad I looked. My hairstyle might provoke head shoving. Her anger persisted for days with anxious morning routines and evenings colored with loud demands and insults. I walked on eggshells until out of nowhere, she was back to normal. It ended as if nothing happened. Once, after tiptoeing around our home for three days, I had to walk forty-five minutes home in the pouring rain because she did not pick me up from band practice as planned. She was in the kitchen when I walked in the door, completely soaked.

"Hey," she said, smiling. "What took you so long?"

"I had to walk home," I replied frustratingly.

"Oh. Okay. Well, dinner is almost ready."

She went back to the pot on the stove. I was too afraid to ask why she didn't come to get me. I did not want to trigger her. She was happy. There was no telling how long it would last.

Explosions were unexpected, particularly when they came in the middle of the night. I was not looking for one on the night before Homecoming. I thought I was hearing voices in a dream. I awoke to Mama, angrily yelling my name.

"Huh?" I mumbled, reaching to turn on the lamp.

"Did you roll your hair?" Her voice was loud.

I glanced at the clock. I was not thinking about my hairstyle at 2:30 a.m.

"Huh," I said again, rubbing my eyes.

"Did you roll your hair?!"

I rolled the back of my hair before I went to bed but wanted the front to be wrapped. Mama had seen me in this hairstyle previously. I explained the style to her. She was not pleased.

"You always do this stupid shit," she screamed from her room. "You like being ugly? That's what you are with your bony, ugly ass. Roll your damn hair before I come in there and knock the hell out of you!"

Tears soaked my cheeks. I opened my desk drawer and reached for a roller. Slowly, I curled the front of my hair around each pink foam. After wrapping my hair with Grandmama's old scarf, I turned the lamp off, put my head on the pillow, and waited for the sun to rise. Tomorrow would be better.

Homecoming 1991. North Charleston High dismissed students early on Friday to prepare for our annual parade. Roaring cheers and whistles traveled through the streets of Liberty Hill back to the old Bonds Wilson parking lot where I stood with the rest of the band. The flagpole held up the weight of my body. Last night was still on my mind despite the bustle of activity around me. People were making final touches to car decorations. ROTC cadets were getting in last-minute practices on their steps. Miss Simmons called us to line up in position. We were set to lead the parade. She reviewed the route. Ever since Bonds Wilson's closure, the route began at the old high school and went through Liberty Hill, through the stoplight, around Park Circle, and finally ending at North Charleston High.

I barely heard the drum major count off because of the cheers from the crowd. We marched down the streets of Liberty Hill. Montague sidewalks were lined with neighbors, parents, and other students. I could see Granddaddy's house on my right as we approached the stoplight. My brother and his friends were yelling my name with pride. I began to feel better about myself and the way I looked. We crossed the intersection and my name echoed again.

"Ruthenna! Ruthenna!"

I gained more confidence with every step. The aftermath of last night's explosion passed. When Mama picked me up after the parade, once again, she acted as if nothing happened. Normal had returned.

David

H omeroom was either a break or fifteen minutes wasted in a high schooler's day. Looking at this girl in my freshman homeroom class was an annoying part of my routine. I hated how my eyes gravitated towards her but I couldn't help it. For some reason, I thought she was the prettiest girl I had ever seen on this side of a television screen. She walked the halls alone most of the time unless she was with him. He was probably the reason I could not take my eyes off her. I often watched her and her boyfriend walking the halls together. At the end of every day, I would run down to my second-floor locker to catch a glimpse of the two of them. Her locker was on an adjacent wall that was in a perfect inconspicuous view for me. So, I watched the pretty white girl with her very black boyfriend.

He was the beauty of this high school relationship. I knew he lived on The Hill. I saw him walking home in the afternoons. There was a swagger in his stride. I curiously watched him walk her to the locker every day. He seemed protective; standing behind her while she gathered her things. The most fascinating thing for me to watch was the way he handled the disapproving stares and offensive remarks. North Charleston High was a predominately black school since the merger. Having a white girlfriend or boyfriend was an anomaly that drew harsh criticism. The maturity with which he silently dismissed ignorance was intriguing. He did not care about the opinions of others. He acknowledged only what he knew to be true in his heart.

I finally met David on a trip to Carowinds Amusement Park in the spring. It was strange to see him without her, but I was relieved. He stood in line with me while I waited to ride roller coasters. I watched him play games for prizes. We laughed and complained about the cost of food. By midday, it felt like a few years passed since we met, though it was just a few hours. There was an effortless familiarity between us that translated to others. Sometimes we were approached by groups of other park goers. They commented on how nice it was for him to bring his girlfriend to Carowinds. Initially, his only response was the same blushing smile he gave me during breakfast. I would quickly correct their assumptions.

"No, no. I'm not his girlfriend," I'd say.

"Oh, is she your sister," one girl asked him?

"I just met him today," I said while he interrupted.

"We're friends," he said with a sly, infectious smile.

One reason others jumped to conclusions was the teddy bear I was holding. He got lucky in one of the basketball game booths. I had not won anything all morning.

"How did you win something so fast?"

He laughed.

"That's not funny," I said jokingly. "I haven't won anything yet. You should give me that one."

David looked at me and smiled. "Why don't you let me win another one? Just for you."

"What if you can't win another one?" I totally missed the flirt.

He thought for a minute.

"Dang. I was gonna give this one to my girl. I promised her I would get her a bear."

"Alright," I said. I heard his integrity. "I get that. You want to win something for her. I'd rather have something meant for me, anyway."

He looked at me with weak eyes.

"Here," he said, giving me the bear. "You look like you don't give up easily. I'll figure something out."

"You don't have to do that."

"No, really. I'll just buy her one. You take this one. So, at least you don't go home empty-handed."

I smiled at him. "Oh, so this is a sympathy bear?"

He smiled back. "Nah, that's definitely not sympathy."

He eventually won another bear later. I wanted to trade but he reminded me how I declined his original offer to win me one of my own. His words were repeated in homeroom on Monday.

The bell rang at the end of the day, and I went to the second floor. She knelt at her locker with the teddy bear. David stood patiently behind her while she gathered her books. She stood and they began to leave. She disappeared into the stairwell, but before leaving my view, he paused and smiled at me. I smiled back, hoping he didn't see me blush. For the next few weeks, I looked for David every day. If I did not see him at school, I hoped to see him on the streets of Liberty Hill. I saw him once, at the end of the school year, while walking home. He smiled at me, releasing the butterflies again.

Summer after freshman year was busy. I worked at a record store and went to band camp every day. There was always a small battle between Miss Simmons and the football coach towards the end of camp. Conflicts over scheduling field time were the usual issue. While they argued, the female band members consciously posed on the field for the football players watching from the bleachers. I was using my flag as a posing prop when I noticed a new, but familiar face sitting with the team. It was no surprise David was a natural athlete. Seeing him in his football jersey was the highlight of every day at band camp. We had not spoken since the trip to Carowinds, and my intrigue had evolved into a full-blown attraction. This was unexplored territory for me. I was not quite ready for emotions so strong.

I decided to deflect my attention towards an easier target. I chose a drummer in the band. Being around him during rehearsals and competitions was a convenient distraction. I imagined us sitting together on bus trips or in the bleachers during band competitions. I never actively pursued this crush, though the drummer was quite aware of it. We often exchanged long glances at each other throughout the day. Reciprocated feelings from him were an afterthought on the first day of my sophomore year.

I saw David as I walked to my third-period class. He was talking with a friend across the hall. I imagined how nice it would be to see him every day, up close on the way to class. We would be closer than I realized. I had already chosen my seat when I saw him walk through my classroom door. I froze. Finally, I would get to know the guy I had watched during my freshman year. This was my chance to discover what made him so intriguing. My chances increased later when he showed up in two more of my classes. The school year looked very promising.

David's girlfriend transferred to another district. I was curious if she had ever been to his house. Neighborhoods like Liberty Hill only saw white people passing through to other destinations in the city. I had some white friends at Buist. Their parents never allowed them to come to my house though I was often invited to theirs. Maybe David's girlfriend was able to stand up for her relationship. When she came to North Charleston for David's birthday, I wondered if her parents knew. David smiled all afternoon when she showed up. I was very jealous. Being in the same classes gave us a lot of time to get to know each other. A close, unexpected friendship was developing. His girlfriend's presence made me afraid friendship was all we would ever have. My fears turned to hope when he told me they broke up before Thanksgiving.

Marching season ended before Christmas, leaving the second semester open for other extracurricular activities. Pageants, contests, and conferences took me all over the country in 1993. Some competitions took me out of school for days.

"How was it?" David asked upon every return.

His thin, slanted eyes looked at me with pride as I told him about the trips and accomplishments. If I failed, he listened and encouraged me. Science was my sophomore struggle. There were mornings I went into third-period class discouraged after receiving a bad Biology grade.

"What's wrong with you," David asked when he sat down before the bell.

My head was down on the desk after nearly flunking my last science test. I did not respond.

"Hey," he tried again.

I refused to lift my head. A second passed and I felt David's hand touch my arm.

"Hey, you alright?"

"Yeah," I slowly responded. "Biology just got me feeling really stupid right now."

"That's bullshit," he said. "You know that, right? You're nowhere near stupid. Come on."

He tried to lift my arm. I believed his words, but I had to wipe my tears.

"Just give me a second."

I could feel his eyes waiting for me to sit up. I raised my head when I heard the teacher's voice. Finally, David turned around to the front of the classroom.

We never discussed the feelings developing between us. On the last day of school, we finally exchanged phone numbers. There were no first-call expectations. We simply labeled the exchange as a normal gesture to keep in touch. One week later, I decided to reach out. I had been thinking about David since the last day of school. I missed seeing him every day and missed our conversations. Lying on my bed on Friday afternoon, I realized according to the clock on my dresser, I would normally be sitting next to him in a classroom. After a lot of jitters and rationalization, I picked up the phone and dialed the number.

I had nothing to be nervous about. He was a little shocked that I called but excited to talk to me. Our phone conversation was like the ones we had in class. We spoke about our first week out of school and summer plans. David decided not to play football. Basketball was his forte. He suggested that we hang out sometime during the summer. I welcomed the idea. It never occurred to me how soon he meant until he called later that evening.

"I wasn't expecting to hear from you for a while," I said.

"Yeah," David replied. "What are you doing?"

"I just got back in the house," I told him how I spent the evening with my big brother.

"Oh. Well, I was wondering if you wanted some company?"

Every inch of my body began to shake.

"You want to come over here? Now?"

He confirmed that I heard him correctly. I was ecstatic. Then, I realized I had to ask Mama, first. I told David to hold on while I asked permission. It was already almost ten o'clock and I had just walked in the door from being with Cole all day. I thought it would be a definite no, but I took a chance. I decided to take the begging route. I walked into Mama's room, pleading.

"Please say yes, Mama. Please say yes."

"Wait, wait, wait. To what?"

I briefly explained my request. She was already familiar with David's family. Everyone knows everyone on Liberty Hill. To my surprise, she did not say no. Her response was still quite strange.

"Call your brother and ask him," Mama replied. "If he says yes, then it's ok."

I did not understand why she wanted me to ask Cole, but I went with the whole thing. I told David to call me right back. I called and paged Cole. He was not home, and he did not respond to my page. After several minutes, Mama agreed to let David come to the house, but I thought her permission was too late. So much time had passed, I was sure David had lost interest. I was wrong.

The phone rang and I answered. I told David the good news but warned him against any future late-night visits. He apologized to me and my mother when he arrived. We sat outside on the porch. The butterflies in my stomach felt like they were going to burst through my pores. Though our conversation was like usual, there was a different aura between us. The air was charged with electricity as if even the slightest touch would cause us to explode. We talked for hours, looking at the stars on that warm Friday night in June. Finally, Mama gave us a thirty-minute warning.

I walked David to his car. As he got in, I battled between disappointment and relief. I wanted my first real kiss that night but shuttered at my inexperience. David closed the door. We joked about our driving skills.

Then he looked up at me and said, "Come here for a second."

I realized what he wanted but I wanted this on my terms.

"No, you come here."

David got out of the car so fast, I backed away to avoid getting hit by him or the door.

"OK, come here," he said as he leaned against the car.

I decided to stall.

"For what," I asked?

He reached for my hand.

"I can't have a kiss or a hug?"

"You can have a hug, but I don't know about a kiss."

I stepped towards him, and we embraced.

"Why not," he whispered?

"You told me I was too friendly, remember?"

"Oh."

We stood embraced for what seemed like an eternity. I had never been held with such sweetness. I could have stayed in his arms for hours, but I was avoiding the inevitable.

I whispered, "Sooo, are you going to stand here all night, waiting for me to kiss you?"

"Nah," he answered. "Only for about three more seconds."

"Oh, really?" He knew how to manipulate my controlling side. "Let's see."

I whispered, "One, two, three."

I pulled away still believing I was not worthy. I lifted my foot slightly, to take a step back, but before I moved, his lips were touching mine. The touch, alone, was enough to make me surrender into the kiss. The ground held up my shaky legs and I followed his lead. The kiss grew longer, and David was gentler. It was sweeter than the embrace. I felt David's heart. I hoped he could feel mine. He made me feel safe. He would never know how he changed a horrible experience for me. David rewrote my first kiss. It was no longer a violation. He returned the innocence that was stolen from an eight-year-old girl.

These Grand Plans

Like many low-income neighborhoods across the country during the '80s and '90s, Liberty Hill became a part of the massive drug trade. Everyone knew someone selling drugs. The dealers were friends, family members, classmates, or old acquaintances. To most of the older generation, the dealers were a bunch of hoodlums with no home training. It was easy to write these young boys off. Discarding what is deemed undesirable is easier than facing the truth.

The truth was many of these young men had home training. A few came from homes filled with love and support. But sometimes, that love and support just wasn't enough when life dealt them a bad hand. It was clear when I learned a classmate started dealing. Monty and I were in the same Honors classes during my freshman year. He was particularly gifted in science. I marveled at his ability to understand formulas and concepts so quickly in our class. I enjoyed watching him learn because he seemed so focused. Though our teacher was not his favorite, Monty listened. His ears seemed to focus through the voice teaching the lesson we were learning and squarely on the information itself. I liked to sneak peeks at his handsome, chiseled face working on class assignments. His intense gaze on the text looked like a genuine interest in the subject; the type that fuels dreams and grows into careers.

Then, in the second semester, Monty's father died. It was unexpected. It was life changing. Monty was understandably absent from school during the ordeal. He returned after a week or so, but then he began to disappear. His attendance turned sporadic. By the end of our freshman year, Monty was gone. I saw him after semester exams while walking home from school. He looked different. He was still the cute guy with caramel skin and wavy hair, but his eyes were darker. I prayed he wouldn't allow his father's passing to rob him of his potential. On The Hill, you're expected to take a licking and keep on ticking. The truth is, sometimes, that's just not possible. It wasn't long before word got out that Monty was selling drugs. A bright and gifted student became another street dealer.

North Charleston High was not immune to the drug infestation of the '90s. A major news story broke when the police raided someone's locker and found a substantial amount of cocaine. The halls were filled with cameras and reporters. Our assistant principal asked if I wanted to be interviewed from a student's perspective. I jumped at another opportunity to be on television. I went on about how sad it was for something like this to happen at our school. I talked about how the student body was so shocked and hurt by the events. I gave the press an intelligent, young, black girl and a whole bunch of crap.

No one was shocked at what the police found. We were shocked they found it, period. Several fellow students were dealing, but I never saw anything done at school. I saw the real deals on my walk home. Liberty Hill's street corners were major markets for small-time hustlers. Many of the guys on the corners were boys who grew up with me. I waved as I passed them walking to someone's car for a pick-up. They always waved back with a loud, "Wassup!"

I was never afraid to walk through my neighborhood. Everyone knew me. Everyone also knew my brother. Cole was known in the street by his first name. Being his little sister was a bit of a shield from violent business disputes. I knew my brother was dealing drugs on a different level than the guys I saw on the corners every day. He was middle management. His money was made crossing borders for the supply. I never saw him making deals, but I heard the phone calls and saw his beeper buzz all the time. He talked about his trips to Florida. He even took me to the gun range and taught me how to shoot.

Like other drug dealers, Cole had a severely flawed plan. The goal was to make enough money to eventually stop dealing and finish his degree. There was only one problem: excessive spending. Cole was accustomed to instant gratification. That ended when Grandmama died. Granddaddy was not as quick to say yes to Cole's request as he was with Mama's. He wanted to teach him the reward of hard work, but Cole was too old and too stubborn to learn the difference between what is entitled in life and what must be earned. It led to constant bad choices.

Though his bad choices angered me to my soul, spending time with my brother was a jewel. He loved me with a swelled chest full of pride. I loved being around his confidence. Cole owned every room he walked into with a charming façade. He dressed in the latest trends with a sophisticated swagger. Young women were drawn to his wide smile and sweet talk. I studied the way he convinced girls to buy him clothes and jewelry. He boldly told them what he wanted while playfully suggesting they should get it for him. Each girl laughed at his audacity but within weeks, Cole had whatever he desired from her. Saying no to him was a difficult feat.

It was near impossible for me to object when my brother brought me bags of crack rocks to hide. We formed a sibling bond against Mama's wrath. He shielded me from her strikes when he was around. A blind trust grew in my heart, allowing me to rationalize stashing little sandwich bags of drugs for him. We hid the bags in stuffed toys. I discreetly placed each stuffed animal back on my bed. Cole would come back for them later. The drugs were never there for more than a few days. I checked the toys daily to see when my brother removed the bags. Though I never really pondered the dangers, I always breathed a sigh of relief when the toys were empty.

Our entire family knew Cole was selling drugs. He received numerous warnings about his lifestyle. Many of his acquaintances were arrested. Friends reminded him of the dangerous consequences. Nothing got through to him. The idea of jail or getting killed was not enough to scare him. Cole believed he was smarter than the system and everyone else around him. He was determined to see this idiotic plan through to the end.

I was with David when I saw Cole at home for the last time. David and I were hanging out on yet another Friday night in November. When Mama told Cole I had company, he rushed over to our house. He was surprisingly civil to David. I enjoyed seeing my big brother be protective. Having Cole meet the boy I cared about was special. After a few minutes, Cole's beeper distracted him. I took that time to get David out while the getting was still good. Mama and Cole were talking when I came back inside from the cold November air. We laughed together and made holiday plans. Those plans should not have included my brother.

The halls of North Charleston High filled with excitement as Thanksgiving grew closer. Football was over and we eagerly awaited the first basketball game of the season. Basketball was North Charleston's pride. With an array of talented players like Virgil Stevens and Jerald Freeman, our team was almost impossible to beat that year. We usually went deep into state playoffs, but the season always began with the Sweet Sixteen Tournament. Our inevitable opponent would be our biggest rival of over thirty years, Burke High School.

This rivalry was legendary. It was part of the legacy brought over from Bonds Wilson High during the merger. Bonds Wilson was a high school built within South Carolina's so-called Equalization program for black students in the 1950s. It was the state's cover to avoid school desegregation. Burke was the largest high school for black students in the downtown Charleston area. There was a treasured competitive history. The games between the two schools were so infamous, Mama still spoke about them from her high school days, almost twenty-five years ago. Game night was an event. The competition on the court was high octane. Scores were always close

LIBERATED FROM THE HILL

in the end. Bragging rights were paramount for each school. Expectations were high for both teams.

Decades passed. Bonds Wilson merged with North Charleston, but the atmosphere had not changed. The rivalry between these two predominantly black schools was still strong. Crowds packed the gym. Alumnae sat in the stands to support. Girls wore the latest fashion trends. Guys put a little extra effort into their appearance as well. Walking to concessions was like walking a catwalk for the city to see. This meant I had to look my best for the first rival game of the season. I knew the way to do that was through my brother's closet.

I drove to Granddaddy's house praying Cole would not be home. I wasn't sure how he'd feel about me borrowing his favorite T-shirt, but I had to wear it. I walked in the door and the house was dark. It seemed no one was home until I walked a little further into the darkness and was almost startled. Granddaddy was sitting in the living room with his hand on his head as the armrest barely held him up. I had never seen him like this. He was quiet and weak.

"You alright, Grandaddy?" I asked.

"Yeah, I'm fine."

I felt like it was best to not push. He wasn't going to tell me anything. Our family didn't discuss issues, especially with children. So, I refocused on the task at hand.

"Is Cole home?"

"No, baby. He ain't here." He replied.

"Ok. Well, I'm just gonna grab a shirt. Please tell him I promise to bring it back."

"Alright."

I went back to Cole's room. I turned the light on and stood at the door of his closet. Something felt weird. Something was wrong, but I couldn't put my finger on it. I opened the door and grabbed the deep red Mickey Mouse T-shirt I came for. The feeling was more specific as I walked back through the dark house. There was a feeling

68

of finality to taking the shirt. I pushed the feelings aside and went to the game. North Charleston won.

A few days after Thanksgiving, Mama came into my room. She was obviously nervous as she told me we needed to talk. I recognized the tone in her voice. This was the same tone in which she told me about Grandmama.

"Did you see the news on Friday? About the big drug bust?" she asked.

I vaguely remembered something about it. She was stalling again.

"Maybe, I'm not sure," I replied.

"Baby. They got your brother." She waited for a response.

"What happened?"

"They caught him at the airport. He had a couple of kilos on him."

I knew that was a lot.

"So, he's in jail?"

"Yeah, baby. He's in jail."

"When will he get out?"

Mama explained about bail hearings and other legal things I did not understand. Only one other question ran through my head as she spoke. I glared at the tiger puppet on my bedpost. What was I supposed to do with the bag inside?

I was not shocked or sad to hear about Cole's bust. A small part of me knew it was coming sooner or later. Cole was reckless at times. Surely, this spilled into his drug deals in some way. I asked God to protect him. I prayed for God to get Cole out of the game. I was almost relieved Cole got caught. At least he wasn't dead. Maybe, a little jail time would be a reality check. Unfortunately, it would be far longer than we hoped.

***

Cole rang in the New Year while sitting in a Charleston County jail cell. Mama and I often did the holidays separate from Granddaddy and Cole. They usually spent Christmas with whatever female tickled their fancy. We spent the day with my Aunt Barbara and Miss Mable. Aunt Barbara was Granddaddy's oldest daughter from his first marriage. She was caring but very intimidating. Miss Mable was one of Grandmama's oldest and dearest friends. She was a strong pillar for Mama after Grandmama died. I spent many days at her house after school. She assumed the grandmother role in my life, as she did for many families on Liberty Hill.

I returned to school in the New Year, wearing my new clothes and the watch David gave me for Christmas. Competitions took a backseat to college preparation as junior year progressed. Though my grades were only a little above average, the advanced-level classes made them look impressive. My extensive list of awards and extracurricular activities helped soften my less-than-perfect GPA. College brochures were coming in the mail every week.

I had no intentions of going to a university in South Carolina. This was my chance to get the hell off Liberty Hill. I dreamed of the college life I saw on episodes of A Different World. Scenes included me at the diner and in dorm rooms. I imagined myself walking around campus from class to class. I saw myself cheering in the stands with sorority sisters. College life was the next stop past the railroad tracks. The excitement motivated me every day of the second semester.

It was important for me to go to a college that exuded the same spirit as North Charleston High. I wanted to feel the pride I saw when I watched the NCAA basketball tournament every year. The schools competing were synonymous with athletes as well as academics. I set my sights on large universities that were basketball powerhouses. I received an Open House invitation from Duke University, but the annual tuition was like a middle-class salary. This sparked my hatred for Duke which still burns in me to this day. Numerous other schools were more budget-friendly. I began looking at wonderful institutions like UNC Chapel Hill and Georgia Tech University.

College was going to be the best thing for me, as well as the very strained relationship with Mama. The way we related to each other began to change as time passed. The beatings dwindled but conversations between us were awkward. Her eyes were fixed and glazed when we tried to talk about my interests. Some of this was the normal environment of having a teenager in the house. Mostly, it was this grown woman living with a strange young lady. I was growing into someone who Mama had no real concept of, and I wondered if this scared her. She wanted what was best for me, but time was flying by. I was ready to leave home and she knew it.

My schedule took me out of the house often. From competitions to social events, I was always on the move. Mama allowed me to use her car after receiving my license. I drove the Buick to school once or twice a week at the beginning of junior year. Then extra-curricular activities increased, and basketball season started. I constantly asked Mama to use her car. By Christmas, she was tired of me asking. We started looking at cars after New Year's. I could not believe Mama was willing to entertain the idea. She, Willie, and I looked around used car lots for two months. I began to lose hope until Mama said she was open to a new car as long as it was cheap. We went to a Hyundai dealership on Valentine's Day. After test driving a cute, red, two-door Excel hatchback, I was sold. Willie and I drove her Buick home while Mama stayed to do the paperwork. As soon as she got back, we sat down to discuss the rules.

We talked about the independence attached to having a car which led to a discussion about the independence coming with me leaving for college soon. With only a little over a year left together, we agreed our relationship would not be the kind where the mother and daughter are best friends. We could, however, make this last year bearable. I didn't want our relationship to end up like hers and Cole's. Mama loved her children, but she just didn't know how to

71

show it. I didn't know how to receive it. This, along with her mental illness, was the root of our problems. Talking through our issues helped us make a pact for my quickly approaching senior year. Both of us agreed to make an effort to get along with each other. We wanted to look back and treasure our last year in the house together.

We decided to begin touring schools in the middle of the second semester of my junior year. The first stop was the University of North Carolina at Charlotte (UNCC). My youth pastor's sister-in-law attended this school. She invited me to spend my spring break with her. My church planned a trip to Disney World during the same week. Mama and I decided I would check out UNCC then fly to Orlando to join the rest of the youth ministry. While I was enjoying my Spring Break, Mama would be in Alabama visiting family. Then we would return with stories about our trips and a resolve to implement the pact we made before leaving. It would be a fresh start.

Rev. Crump and his wife, Dawn, were going to drive me to Charlotte on Friday of my Spring Break. They were patiently waiting when I darted through the back door. The hairdresser had taken forever on my hair. Thankfully, I packed the night before. Rev. Crump opened the car door for Dawn and placed my suitcase in the trunk. I gave Mama a big hug.

"I'll call you when I get to Alabama. Y'all be safe on that road," Mama said.

"You, too," I replied. "You drive safely."

"Ok. I love you."

"I love you too."

I got in the car and waved as we pulled out of the driveway. Mama waved back. She was standing with the door open and a smile on her face. I waved until she was out of sight.

Mama and I spoke briefly while I was in Charlotte. We were enjoying ourselves in separate locations. She sent regards from our cousins in Alabama. I told her my thoughts on UNCC. I liked the school, but I loved the city. Charlotte was hosting the 1994 NCAA

Final Four Basketball Tournament. Surrounded by a reality I had only seen on television made my dreams seem possible. Mama could hear the excitement in my voice. We exchanged loving sentiments, said goodbye, and hung up. That was the last time I spoke to Mama.

After a few days, I flew to Orlando as planned. The next Friday, the group returned, and I went home with our youth advisor, Raquel. She was the jewel of youth ministry at our church. The Earth could never hold the love she had for the kids at Abundant Life. She often went to school to advocate for us. She introduced many of us to college life with trips and tours. Raquel was a bridge between our feelings and the ears of our parents. She was our rock. Spending time with her was common for many of us at church. Since Mama was not coming home until Sunday, I stayed with Raquel until then.

I was not shocked when Mama didn't show up on Sunday evening. This was not the first time she did this. Times and days got confused or something came up. I spent the night with Raquel. The next morning, I called home but there was no answer. Raquel took me to school. I was not worried as I walked into my first class. When the lunch bell rang, I went to the crowded courtyard. Everyone was sharing spring break stories. I told my friends about my trips. Reviewing the week made me wonder how Mama got any details confused.

By the end of the day, I was concerned. I went to one of the payphones in school and called home. Still, no answer. I decided to use the phone card Mama gave me, to call our cousins in Alabama. I was concerned, but they were frantic. Mama got on the road the day before, on April 10, 1994. She was supposed to call them when she got home from the eight-hour drive. It was April 11 and I was calling them instead. I walked home from school. Mama's old car sat in the driveway, but the new hatchback she used for the trip was still gone. I used my keys to open the house door.

I waited for Mama to come home. It never occurred to me that she wouldn't. Several hours passed when finally, I heard someone at the door. I looked through the peephole into my stepfather's eyes. He came in and I told him about the last twenty-four hours. I called Alabama again, only to hear the same news. They still had not heard from her. Willie's eyes glazed over with worry. For the first time, I was genuinely scared. We sat in my room with no idea what to do. The time was nearing 10 p.m.

One of Mama's best friends, Deborah, called to speak with her. I told her what was going on. She asked for a few details and told me she would call back. I felt a little relief in knowing someone else was offering help. Only a few minutes passed before she called back.

"Quala, your mom was in an accident."

I listened to the little information she was able to obtain from the State Patrol. Mama was in a hospital in Macon, Georgia. She had been there since Sunday afternoon. Deborah called the hospital but was not able to get much from them because she was not family. She gave me the number. I called the hospital. I told the nurses who I was and asked to speak to Mama. The hospital staff said I couldn't speak with her either. They explained she was on life support machines and unable to talk. I listened a bit more, then hung up the phone.

Willie said to call Granddaddy and Aunt Barbara immediately. I called Granddaddy first and then Aunt Barbara. To my surprise, they were already aware of the events. In the last twenty-four hours of my emotional roller coaster of concern, the two of them made a trip to Georgia the day before. They had seen Mama, spoken with doctors, and made decisions about her care. They spent the night and returned earlier that afternoon. They did all of this, and I had no clue. Barbara told me how tired they were. I called when she was just about to go to bed. She said she needed her rest and did not feel the need to talk anymore. She said goodbye and hung up.

I sat silently with Willie. The silence screamed all my questions. How did Willie and I fit into the equation? When were they planning on telling us what happened? No one thought to call the school? Why

74

didn't they call the house to check on me? Did they even wonder where I was? A call back from my aunt quickly reminded me what priorities were in my maternal family. My well-being took second place to appearances. Barbara sternly advised me to go stay with Granddaddy. She felt it would not look right for a sixteen-year-old to stay in the house where I grew up, with the man who helped raise me since age six. Willie did not argue. I hated his complacent attitude with my family.

We drove to Raquel's house to get my things. I told her about the accident. She was a nurse which helped give perspective on the possibilities of Mama's condition. We went back to the house where I packed a few things to go to Granddaddy's.

"This is not right," I said. "We don't have to do this. I should just stay with you in the house. This is stupid."

"We gotta do what your aunt said, Quala."

I was furious. This scenario was painfully familiar. A few years earlier, when a friend of Mama's passed away, the kids were forced to stay with relatives instead of with the man, Jake, whom they knew as their father. For months, they repeatedly ran away to their loving Jake, only to be sent back to relatives they were forced upon. They were not allowed to be with the only other parent they knew, the other person who loved them in the way they desperately needed at the most difficult time of their lives. Now, it was happening to me. I suddenly felt their pain and fear.

I went to Granddaddy's house that night. I was not happy, but thought, surely, this would be a temporary situation. I chose to look ahead with positivity. Mama was not going to die. She would get better. She would come home. We would start fresh just like we planned. Right?

Loss

Tubes were coming out of every hole in Mama's body. Needles were in both arms. Half of her head was shaved. Her right leg was in a cast hanging from a sling connected to a metal pole over the bed. The left leg lay limp like an old doll's limb. Her face was swollen to the size of a basketball with her eyes closed. Scrapes and bruises covered her hands and arms. The beeping from the heart monitor was loud, and the sound of the ventilator breathing oxygen into her mouth was almost offensive. It was a slow, hard release of air, filling her lungs and suffocating the room.

I stood at the door of the hospital room for about five minutes. The doctor warned me she would appear worse than her improving condition. Mama was breathing on her own for thirty-six hours. The ventilator was a precautionary measure as well as for monitoring purposes. Nurses shaved one side of her head just before emergency brain surgery when she arrived five days earlier. I could see a small piece of the scar peeking from the end of the bandage covering where the incision on her skull was made. The operation was successful in stopping the bleeding on her brain. Her leg underwent surgery as well.. The cast protected the broken bones and assisted healing.

The hospital room was dimly lit but I could see her swollen face. As I watched her chest rise and fall, my mind began to wonder. After severe verbal lashings from Mama, I often fantasized about being raised by someone else. This felt eerily close to the dramatic scene I created in my head. In a surprise twist for my family, Mama's pastor would be called to the reading of her will and there would be a clause regarding my custody. Shock consumed the entire attorney's office as the lawyer announced the pastor was my new guardian. He would be reluctant at first but settle into the idea as time passed. I would live in his big house for a few years. His family would accept me as one of their own. Then, after graduation, I would head off to college to start life as an adult.

Standing in Mama's hospital room, I felt like I was at the cusp of this fantasy. I searched her face, but I did not see death. She was not going to die. Finally exhaling, I opened the door and walked out. It wasn't a scene from a movie, this was very real. My feelings didn't make sense as I walked down the hall. I wasn't sad or scared. There was no guilt or disappointment at the absurdity of the fantasy. I was numb. An unseen fog swallowed my feet like quicksand. My pace was slow. My steps, unsure.

Later that evening I laid in the bed of a cheap motel room. Barbara, Granddaddy, and I spent the night in Macon, Georgia to rest before the four-hour drive back home the next day. I hated that room. I mostly hated being in the room with them. What did they think when they got the call about Mama's accident? Did they even ask if I was with her? Three nights ago, my aunt and my grandfather slept while I was awake waiting for Mama to come home. They slept in the same manner while I lay awake in unfamiliar loneliness.

A small glimpse of the hospital appeared in the distance through the motel room window. I wondered how Mama was sleeping and I suddenly found myself missing her. It made me want to go to her room and get in the comfort of her bed as I did on nights when I was afraid of my dreams. Our fights did not matter on those nights. The sting of her hand and the pain of her words always shrank in the face of my need for the security of her presence. I could not wait to see her as the sun rose the next morning.

Two days later, I made a second trip to Macon, Georgia when I had a chance to meet the couple who saved Mama's life. That Saturday, Willie's sister, Auntie Liz, rented a car for us to go see Mama. Miss Mable joined us for the trip. To my dismay, so did Barbara. I was grateful for Auntie Liz's presence. Auntie Liz held a reserved wisdom about her that deemed her the matriarch of Willie's family. She understood the solace I found in being in my Mama's presence. Nicole, her 10-year-old daughter, came too. Six people packed into a two-door coupe for a four-hour drive.

When we arrived at the hospital, we were directed to a different room. Mama was off the machines and breathing on her own. She went through a second surgery on her head. The swelling on her brain decreased, which allowed her to be transferred out of the trauma unit. As we approached her room, a slender white woman greeted us in the hallway.

"You must be her daughter!" She said, smiling at me.

I loved her immediately. For the first time in the last six days, I felt acknowledged. She gave me a warm, gentle hug. This was the angel I was waiting to meet. Sera and her husband, Gabriel, witnessed another car hit Mama's vehicle as it passed at a high speed. The car never stopped. They saw Mama's vehicle flip three times before she was thrown out of the hatchback. Upon impact her epilepsy was triggered, prompting multiple seizures. The couple stayed with Mama until the ambulance arrived. They visited her every day on the days we could not make the trip down to Georgia.

"I didn't know you were coming," Sera said.

Barbara met Sera with Granddaddy when they came on the day of the accident. She made introductions. All six of us spoke with her for a few minutes before going to Mama's room.

Mama was awake, though she could barely speak. I read the desperation for mobility in her clenched hands. Her relief to see loving and familiar faces glimmered in the tear sliding out the corner of her eye to the pillow. She smiled. I hurt for Mama. How scared was she when she woke up the first time and did not see anyone she knew for days? I walked over and took her hand. Soon, Mama drifted off to a place between sleep and unconsciousness. I gently removed her hand from mine and placed it on the bed. I looked at her face once more, then walked to a corner of the room to look out the window.

Auntie Liz quietly sat in a chair with Nicole on her lap. I looked at them and longed for the love my little cousin received from her momma. She was only a few years younger than me, but I learned you are never too big to be held by your mother. My head turned when I heard groans from the bed. Mama was still asleep but it seemed she was trying to say something.

"Sandra." Barbara called to her.

Mama did not respond. She was quiet then she began to chuckle a bit. It was faint. A smile formed on her face and the shape of her eyes changed. Her eyelids tightened. The smile was gone. She opened her mouth to speak. Her words were clear.

"Oh. Oh no! Oh shit! Oh shit!" Then there was nothing.

Everyone looked at the bed. We were silent as we realized what was happening. We had just seen a glimpse of the accident. We got a peek into her fear and panic.

"I'm gonna go outside," Auntie Liz said as she stood up and walked Nicole to the door.

I followed them out of the room.

"Are you ok?" I asked.

"Yeah. I just can't handle all that. That's too much. And Nicole don't need to see that."

"Yeah," I replied.

"But you go ahead. Go in there and be with yo' Momma."

I gave her a very small grin, turned, and walked back to the room. Mama opened her eyes a few more times before we left. I hated leaving her there alone. I took comfort knowing Sera and Gabriel would check on her as often as possible. I called them when I was missing Mama. The sweet-spirited wife gave me updates. She also asked me how I was doing. She asked about school and how I was dealing with everything. Her genuine concern made me feel like someone remembered I was Mama's daughter. She spent three more weeks in the Georgia hospital before being transported to the

Medical University of South Carolina (MUSC) hospital in downtown Charleston.

Meanwhile, life moved on in Liberty Hill. I went to school. Willie and Barbara went to work. Granddaddy dealt with Cole's case. The judicial process was moving swiftly. Only a few weeks passed before Granddaddy went to my brother's sentence hearing. That May afternoon was the first time I saw Granddaddy cry since Grandmama's funeral. I came back from school to find him sitting in a chair in the living room. The air in the room was so heavy. His large stature was weakened with sadness. The chair's armrest supported his worn, blackened elbow. The only thing keeping his head up was his wrinkled hand.

"I went to the courthouse today. They gave your brother 25 years."

The tears fell from Granddaddy's face.

"There was nothing I could do. I just…" He tried.

I stood there and watched this man sink. His daughter was in the hospital. His grandson, who he considered his son, was going to prison. I was there but my presence was irrelevant to him. Granddaddy needed consolation I was incapable of giving. My gut told me Cole would not serve the full time. It was similar to the feeling telling me Mama was not going to die. I wanted to tell my grandfather or reach out to hold him. But our family did not express affection in this way. So, I said the only thing that came to mind.

"I'm sorry, Granddaddy."

I was so sorry. I was sorry Cole had given him so much trouble for the last few years. I thought about the horrible ways he treated the man he called "Daddy." The worst was the day he called Granddaddy "a crippled punk" as he sat in a wheelchair recovering from cancer treatment. My grandfather continuously forgave my brother for his constant disrespect. Cole was given every opportunity our grandparents could afford. Somehow, he managed to waste every single one. I hated the helplessness I saw that afternoon.

Granddaddy loved Cole. Love fueled his belief in Cole's potential. My brother was intellectually smart. He excelled at computer technology. He could have been quite successful, but all of that potential would sit in a prison cell. My grandfather mourned a young man he would never see.

Cole slept in a prison cell while I slept in his bedroom. It felt like a weird sleepover, nothing like the weekends I spent with Grandmama when I was younger. The house was brighter then. Aromas of her mouth-watering breakfasts and delicious dinners traveled down the halls to meet you. Sounds of soap operas and game shows filled different rooms. Now, the house was silent. It was void. Each room felt as suffocating as the room where the ventilator forced oxygen into Mama's body. There was nothing natural about me being there. I was not comfortable. I was not home.

Miss Mable's house became a new place of comfort for me. I began spending more time there after school and on weekends, when we returned from our trip to Georgia. I breathed easier in her house. Eating her cooking took me back to sitting at Grandmama's kitchen table. They both knew their way around a stove, although Miss Mable's meals tended to be a little spicier, like her personality. I loved eating her crispy, oven-baked fish. It reminded me of early morning fishing trips with her and Grandmama when I was younger. Memories of them teaching me how to bait the hook and hold the line were still vivid. I missed Grandmama. It is one of the reasons I liked going to Miss Mable's. Her house was a piece of home I longed for.

School was another place where I could breathe. I enjoyed the extra independence the circumstances provided. Life with minimal supervision is a dream for a 16-year-old. I drove myself to school every day. I drove myself to take the SATs. I prepared college applications while picking my senior year classes. No one asked where I went on Saturday mornings when I left for my weekly scholars' program. Wearing a crown was still a dream I pursued with two pageants approaching. Since the WPAL radio station pageant was not scheduled until the summer, I focused on one pageant at a time.

Preparations for the Miss North Charleston High pageant began before the accident. Mama took me to the library to check out *On the Pulse of Morning* by Maya Angelou. I wanted to recite a portion of the poem for my talent. We decided to use an evening gown from a previous pageant. She was supposed to take me shopping for casual wear when she returned from Alabama. Since shopping with her was no longer possible, I decided to use one of my favorite stylish outfits for the competition and have my big sister, Tasha, do my hair.

The night of the pageant, I went to Mama's house to get ready. I gathered everything I needed, neatly hanging the outfits and gown in a garment bag. I packed my shoes, curling irons, and bobby pins. Then, I froze. Something was missing. I looked around before sitting on my bed. Then, it occurred to me. Some*thing* wasn't missing, it was some*one*. Mama was missing. This was the first event in my life where she would not be there to support me. I was accustomed to her presence. Though many of her insults came before I would go on stage, she always exuded pride after every performance. I always felt her love in the end. A loud knock snapped me into the present before the tears fell. Tonight, the love and pride of my Stepdaddy would have to do.

The next day, I went to visit Mama at MUSC. Mama was awake most days. Her hair was growing back on the right side of her head. The hair on the other side was straight and four inches long. She had lost several front teeth. Her leg was still in a cast. She was much thinner, even for her signature small frame. All of this was expected, but her aura was different. There was nothing maternal about our conversations. Mama seemed younger. Some days I felt like I was speaking to an older woman I happened to know. Other days, she seemed like an acquaintance at school. Every time I visited Mama, the woman in the hospital bed felt less and less familiar.

I liked going to visit her alone. It felt like the only time I had my Mama to myself. At first, I sat in her hospital room with hope and anticipation for when we both could go home. I noticed a difference in her after a couple weeks. One afternoon, I went to her room excited to tell her about a good grade I received.

"Look, Mama," I said, showing her my test.

"Um-hmm," she responded.

I looked at her face. There was no pride. There was no emotion. I pushed it off on the medication or her being tired.

Another day, I came and one of the nurses stopped me before I went in to see Mama. The nurse was kind but looked very serious.

"Let me warn you before going in. We had to restrain your mother."

"Why?" I asked.

"She's been trying to get up and pulling at her IV. She just really wants to go home," the nurse explained. I saw the bands around her wrists as soon as I walked into the hospital room. Her hands were gently but securely tied to the bed rail.

"Hey." She motioned for me to come over with her finger.

I walked to the side of the bed.

"I need you to take these off," she whispered.

"I can't."

"Yes, you can. Just untie 'em."

"I'm not going to take them off. They're for your own good," I told her.

"I'm yo' momma, right?"

Was she asking me about this? I was confused.

"Yes, ma'am."

"Then do what the fuck I'm telling you to do and take this shit off!"

The words sounded like the old verbal beatings but different. I didn't have to take this lashing.

"Okay," I said. "I can't stay here for this." I got up to leave.

"Well, fuck you!"

The statement stopped me in my tracks. I turned around and looked at her. She had already turned her head towards the TV. I walked out of the room. Mama said that to Cole, but she never said it to me. Even at her worst, she never cursed me with what seemed like hatred. When I got to her car, I sat in the driver's seat for a few minutes. *What in the world just happened?*

The Last Summer Begins

Y eah. She drove to the beach. She got out of her car. She put on her headphones to listen to her favorite band. Then she pulled out a gun and shot herself."

My heart dropped as I held the phone in my hand. I listened to K'Lani tell me how one of our middle school classmates, Leah, killed herself.

"Did anyone know anything was wrong?" I asked.

"I'm not sure. Emily didn't know too many details." She replied. There were plenty of hindsight speculations but at the end of the day, no one saw it coming.

Leah filled my thoughts as I hung up the phone. Three years had passed since we saw or spoke to each other at our eighth-grade commencement ceremony. We were not close, but I really liked her. She never joined in with the other classmates who bullied me at Buist and laughed at my expense. She was nice. Most of the other middle school girls were boy crazy and clothing obsessed, but not Leah. She always seemed unfazed by the chaos around her. That's one of the reasons I was so shocked by her suicide.

I needed to talk with an adult about her. Granddaddy sat on the sofa across from me while I heard the news from K'Lani. His 76-year-old wisdom seemed necessary at the time. I walked over to sit next to him and explained what happened to my former classmate.

He barely looked at me when he said, "Hm Hm Hm. That's a shame."

His monotone response matched the fixed eyes on his unmoved face. Maybe I didn't express how this was affecting me.

"Leah was a nice girl," I explained. "She was always so kind to me."

Granddaddy stared out the window.

"We were the same age," I continued. "Now, she's not even going to graduate high school."

He didn't respond. My classmate meant nothing to him. I wondered if he cared that she meant something to me. A minute later, Granddaddy looked up. His silent gaze pierced through my eyes to reveal the truth. I did not care as much as I was curious.

I was curious about the strength it must have taken to say, "The hell with it!" Somehow, I saw bravery in her ability to pull the trigger. The idea was mesmerizing; her standing on the overlook, watching the waves as the long, brown hair I envied in middle school, swayed in the sea breeze. It made sense to have her favorite band playing in her ears at the end. She needed to hear something to help facilitate what she was about to do.

I wondered what song she listened to and what lyrics were playing. The questions ran through my mind as Granddaddy left me alone on the sofa. I looked around my grandparents' living room. I was in this house for two months while Mama was in the hospital. Listening to music in this house felt awkward. I did not appreciate the beautiful melodies and poetic lyrics the way I did at home, in my room, on my stereo. Though Cole's room was at the back of the house, I always felt like playing music disturbed Granddaddy. So, I played nothing.

Charleston County transferred Cole to Lieber Correctional Institution. He was Inmate 211771. I was finally able to speak with him when he received phone privileges. Every conversation lasted until the imposing beep, warning his twenty minutes were almost up. Sometimes, the calls cut off right before he would endearingly say, "Love you, Brat."

I was happy to hear his voice. My brother always tried to make me feel protected. That did not change when he went to prison. Cole called a few times a week. He asked how I was doing. We talked about my approaching senior year and upcoming pageant. Cole was eager to hear what was happening outside of prison walls and I was eager to tell him. My brother seemed to be the only family member interested in my life. I also figured the phone calls were the highlight of his day. But those highlights were costly.

Inmates can only call collect, and each call was around $9. Granddaddy's phone bill was almost $40 more than usual, even if Cole only called once a week. Granddaddy accepted all of the calls initially. He missed Cole very much. Then the phone bills got higher and higher. Finally, Granddaddy decided to only accept the calls when we were both at home. Later, Cole's phone calls doubled in price. The county took the time limit off, but at nearly $18 each, those calls were a luxury. Conversations with Cole were valuable to me. Talking to my brother seemed to soothe the nagging and growing ache of loneliness in my soul.

School was also good medicine. Walking the halls of North Charleston High was the only familiar aspect of my life. I could be myself. I looked forward to the routine of classes, lunch, and seeing my friends. There were a lot of people I hung out with but there were three girls with whom I spent most of my social time. We met during those sweltering days of band camp. All three played clarinet and were a grade behind me. Shelly, Trena, and Lisa were affectionately called my Crew. I was the only person with a driver's license and access to a car, so I always steered the ship.

We were all born and raised on Liberty Hill, although Trena claimed The Hike or Charleston Heights as her original home. We lived a short walk away from each other. The crew was my first call on the night Mama brought the new car home. We rode to school together the next day and almost every morning until Spring Break. Those rides stopped after the accident. Living at Granddaddy's house changed my morning routine. I made time to drive the crew home from school occasionally. The last day of my junior year was a special occasion

The parking lot filled with activity as smiling students poured out of the school after the last bell rang. I loved the sounds of laughter and seeing the relief on people's faces. There always seemed to be a large, unified exhale on the last day of school. For juniors, the day felt a little different. The last summer as a high school student presents a finality to a teenager that is a bit scary. The next summer as a high school graduate comes with new responsibilities and expectations. For me, it felt like I was hitting this milestone a year too early with my mother scheduled to be discharged from the hospital the next day. Her release consumed my mind all morning. I walked out to the school parking lot and took a deep breath. I was still holding it when I heard a familiar voice.

"Hey!" Shelly yelled. Her voice was authoritative.

We carried a similar shell of strength that enabled us to function in the face of our peers. No one knew the struggles or insecurities we masked with our talents and competitive natures.

"Hey Girl," I yelled back. "Where's Trena? Oh, wait."

Trena walked up to us with her usual ponytail and smile. She was the sweet one of the crew. Trena didn't say much but when she did, she kept us laughing. I think we always underestimated her. She unconsciously hid how sharp she was. Or, maybe Trena was smart enough to know what to share and what to keep to herself.

Lisa caught up with us as we walked to the car. It was a beautiful day and only a little after 11 a.m.

"Do y'all feel like going home right now," I asked?

"No, not really," Shelly replied.

"So, what do y'all wanna do?" Lisa was usually up for anything.

A few seconds passed before the light bulb went off in my head. "Oooo. Let's go to Burke!"

Lisa's face lit up. "Yeah! Let's go to Burke."

The idea of going to our rival school sounded so exciting to our teenage ears. Seeing fresh faces would be a welcome change and something different.

"Wait! Don't they get out at 11:00 today too?" Trena asked. She was always the voice of reason in our group.

"I don't know," I said. "Let's just go see."

I didn't care what time they got out. I just wanted to go anywhere other than my grandfather's house.

We got in Granddaddy's white Chrysler Lebaron. He made me stop driving Mama's car a few weeks after I started living with him. It was like Mama was being taken from me, piece by piece. I hated it. I was still grateful to be driving.

We pulled off and headed downtown towards our rival school. I knew a lot of people there from my years at Buist. My best friend, K'Lani, was a student at Burke as well. She was the first person I looked for when we arrived. We got such a rush walking around the school's sprawling campus. We wondered if someone would spot us as outsiders, but we fit right in. We had a little fun seeing people we knew. I found K'Lani and we went back to the car. After a while, I took everyone home, but I still was not ready to go back to Granddaddy's house. So, I went home too.

I walked through the back door of Mama's house and exhaled the breath I was holding since the school bell rang. I missed the beautiful mauves and crèmes in the living room. I missed the tile Willie lovingly and skillfully laid throughout the house. I missed my bedroom. I missed the gray carpet Mama and Willie surprised me with after I returned from a sleepover. I missed the stereo they gave me for Christmas one year. I missed all of my books and cassette tapes. I sat on my bed and for the first time, the tears came pouring down my cheeks. Mama was getting out of the hospital tomorrow, and I would not be able to bring her here. She did not know this place. She did not know me.

Each day I visited Mama, I could see something was not right. There was something unfamiliar about me to her. I felt it. She did not show the same happiness when I walked into the hospital room, as she did when it was Granddaddy or Barbara. Later, I learned Mama had lost about half of her memory. She knew who she was, but a huge chunk of time was gone. She had no recollection of

Grandmama's death or her relationship with Willie. She remembered giving birth to Cole but had no idea he was in jail. To her, he was still a baby. As for me... I was a complete stranger.

My first day of summer started in the hospital. I sat in the nurses' office while they explained instructions for Mama's care. Though she was being released, her recovery was far from over. A physical therapist and speech therapist would come to the house once a week. An occupational therapist would come twice a week. There would also be weekly visits from a nurse. A social worker would come by twice a month to discuss assistance with home health care agencies and other programs. A tube was attached to Mama's stomach to ensure she received the necessary nutrition on days she didn't eat enough. Her appetite would not be normal for several weeks.

Before releasing her, they showed me how to use the tube properly. I held the tube at a slight angle and slowly poured the liquid supplement into the opening. The important step was not to let the tube overflow. It could cause a blockage leading to a visit to the emergency room. Preventing this simply meant slowly pouring small amounts and stopping periodically to allow the liquid to pass through the tube. Then, I would repeat until either the can was empty or she was full. The hospital provided a week's supply of the supplement. I could purchase the rest at the drug store until the doctor removed the tube.

The list of medications was not long but still extensive. There were two medicines for her epilepsy. I was used to those. Since the age of six, I remembered waking up to the sound of Mama's seizures. They didn't happen often. If she forgot to take her medicine or if she was over-stressed, the night would be quite eventful. I would hear grunts and hiccup noises coming from her room. The sounds of things hitting the floor were loud enough to reach my door.

I would call out, "Mama!"

If she did not respond, I ran to her room. When I turned the light on, she would be convulsing in the bed.

"Mama." I'd call once more hoping she could help me but knew she couldn't.

As long as there was no blood and she was breathing, there was no need to call an ambulance. The only thing to do was to try to turn her on her side and wait it out.

The convulsions usually stopped after about 40 seconds and temporary paralysis occurred. Then the moans would begin. They grew increasingly louder and longer. Since her body could not move, I would go get a wet washcloth and come back. I wiped the saliva from her mouth as she moaned. Then I would fold the cloth and gently wipe my Mama's face. Soon after, her eyes would open. She always looked at me in confusion.

"Mama, you ok?"

I don't think she ever heard me during those times.

Still dazed, she would get up and stagger around the house. I followed close behind, making sure she did not fall. She turned the lights on and off. She opened the fridge. She went into almost every room, scanning for the unknown. Finally, she would go back to her bedroom. I would lay her down and put on her covers. When I was sure she was asleep, I got up to head back to my room. I always stopped at the door.

"I love you, Mama."

Then, I turned off the light and went to my room, slowly drifting back to the usual light sleep.

As the nurse explained what to do in case Mama had a seizure, I stopped her.

"I'm very familiar with the process. I grew up with the process." She looked at me.

"Is it just going to be you with her?" The nurse asked. "By yourself?"

"Oh no," I replied. "I'm moving her in with my grandfather. It will be the three of us."

"But," she hesitated, "he's not well either."

91

She was right. Granddaddy was battling bone cancer for a few years. Surgery helped but did not cure the disease. The pain in his legs had flared up again. I took him to the emergency room only a couple of Saturdays before. I woke up that morning and found him still in bed which was very unusual. Granddaddy was an early riser. He was active and loved to be on the go. That morning, he could barely get dressed. He calmly told me he needed me to take him to the doctor. The only problem was he wanted me to drive his truck. It was the only vehicle he felt comfortable enough to ride in with his pain. The truck was beautiful, but it was huge. I was terrified to drive it. The solution was for me to drive to the gate of the George LaGree projects. One of his friends would be waiting there and she would take over the wheel. She drove us to the hospital. They gave him something for the pain and released him. Since that trip, he had one doctor's appointment. The cancer was coming back and slowly eating away at his bones.

"He's managing," I told the nurse.

I saw the concern on her face.

"How old are you?" She asked.

"Sixteen."

She looked me over.

"You know I really should be giving all this to an adult. You're still a minor. Are you sure you can handle all this?"

I shrugged and answered, "I kinda have to. I mean, who else is there?"

"Don't you have any siblings that can help?"

"My brother is in prison. But my aunt is going to help as much as she can."

"That's good, but what about school?" She asked. "What grade are you in?"

"I'll be a senior this year. And since it's the summer, I have all this time to focus on getting my mother better, so we can go home."

The nurse was suspiciously quiet. She smiled sympathetically.

"You know your mom has lost a lot of her memory, right?"

"Yes, I know it's going to take some time, but I'm looking at it as a chance to start over."

There was that look on her face again. I could not decide if her sympathy was annoying or scary.

"That's a good way to look at it," she said. "But the best advice I can give you is don't have any expectations. Your Mom is alive. That's what matters. My mother passed and I miss her all the time. Yours is still here. And she's come a long way. That's something to be thankful for."

I listened to the nurse as she gave advice and more details on home care. I felt a bit overwhelmed. Would I remember all this information? What if I missed something? How long would I have to do all of this? Will I be home by the time school starts? I had so many questions.

My nerves were calmed by the paperwork the nurse gave me, filled with detailed instructions. There were names, phone numbers, steps, and procedures. It was good to know I had something for reference. Weirdly, I felt confident. I always liked the idea of responsibility. I figured this was just another level. The hefty, manila envelope in my hand made me feel prepared as I helped Mama into the car. I pulled off with her in the front seat and Granddaddy in the back. I was not at all prepared for how my life would completely change. I had no clue.

The New Normal

Some kind of shift happened when I walked through the door behind my mother and grandfather. The house I stayed in for the last two months was their home. My Grandfather built this house. Mama was raised in this house. I was a loved but tolerated guest. They went into the living room. Granddaddy turned on the television and joined her on the sofa. I clung to the bulky manila envelope while settling Mama's belongings in her old childhood room. It was converted to a guest room, but the familiarity of her teenage bedroom furniture would be comforting to her. I still held the big envelope as I walked out of the room and back down the hall towards them. Granddaddy's face was brighter sitting next to her. She relaxed on the sofa close to her Daddy. Her eyes were bright with a childhood peace. A little smile, only seen around him, formed on her face. I did not see my Mama sitting on that couch. This was Sammy's daughter.

Joining them in the living room felt like an intrusion. I turned left into the dining room. Sitting down at the table, I took the contents out of the folder. The two were still in my peripheral vision as I read and reviewed all the information. I heard them as I organized the paperwork into other folders. Then, the inevitable question came from her lips.

"Where's Momma?"

I turned to see Granddaddy face his daughter.

"Remember. I told you. She died a few years ago."

"Oh, yeah," she recalled as tears streamed down her face.

Granddaddy and Mama sat quietly, mourning Grandmama's death all over again.

One of the things I was not prepared for was how much work was needed to get Granddaddy's house ready for two sick people. It was not in complete disarray, but it needed a deep and thorough cleaning. Granddaddy had done his best since Grandmama died, but he was from a different generation. He was a man from a time where men worked, and women kept the house in order. My grandmother did it well. After she passed, the house needed a woman's touch.

There was also the matter of the dogs. Granddaddy had two Chihuahuas. Little and Charaka were a part of the family for over a decade. I watched Little lick Charaka off after giving birth to him. When Grandmama died, Charaka howled for days, and Little would not leave the head of the bed where Grandmama slept. They clung to Granddaddy. He loved those dogs. He fed them and cuddled them. I liked the dogs, but I was not used to living with pets. Dogs required a level of care that Mama and I were never willing to give, most specifically, cleaning up after them. This was something my grandfather was very willing to do. Little and Charaka were housebroken but still needed regular baths to prevent fleas. Those baths were much less frequent as age and cancer began to take its toll on Granddaddy's body. The carpets in the house were infested with critters.

Over the past two months, I cleaned as well as a 16-year-old could. This meant a lazy minimum. I swept the carpets because Granddaddy did not have a vacuum. I washed dishes and scrubbed the tub. I did what I felt was my responsibility without being asked. When I brought Mama to her new home, I realized I had to do a lot more. I wanted a fresh house to start this summer of care. But five years passed since the house had received a deep cleaning. The kitchen needed the most work. The floors needed to be scrubbed. Disinfecting the counter was on the list. The fridge needed to be purged along with the atrocious cabinets. It would be an enormous job.

The next day, Sunday, Barbara came by after church. Dressed in a short-sleeved, Hawaiian button-down shirt and shorts, she started cooking. The meal was large enough to last a few days. After

95

cleaning the mess from dinner, she sat down on the sofa by the window.

"So, what did they tell you?" She asked me.

I showed her a few of the documents from the manila envelope. Barbara briefly looked them over. I explained the care instructions the nurse gave and showed her how to feed Mama through the tube in her stomach. Her eyes scanned the living room.

"You go'n have to really clean this house," she said. "It's go'n be a lot of people coming in and out."

My face got hot as Barbara spoke.

She continued, "I can only get here on Sundays after church. You know I'm working all week."

"Yes ma'am," I replied.

"Alright. You need to start here." She said, pointing at the dingy green carpet.

She spewed out her list of things I needed to do in the house. According to her, my top priority, besides care, should be making sure the house was more than presentable. The list, although helpful, felt like an assignment from an onerous boss. There were times Barbara's listening ear provided refuge from Mama's physical and emotional beatings. My aunt was always sympathetic. She reassured me that I was smart, strong, and capable. Now, her words had me overwhelmed.

I woke up Monday morning, with so much on my mind, I could barely think straight. This was the last day before the health care professionals would start showing up. I asked Granddaddy what he needed. I got Mama settled for the day. Then, I walked to the kitchen. Barbara's list replayed in my mind. My list replayed as well. How was I going to get ready? How was I going to do all this work and take care of two people, by myself? The responsibility I thought I would like after leaving the hospital, was closing in on me like walls of a shrinking room. There was no way out. I was just about to panic when I looked through the screen door and saw a small-framed woman coming up the back porch.

"Hey!" she said in that familiar cracked, high pitch voice of hers.

Pine's voice was distinctive but similar to her older sister, Auntie Mina. Alberta "Pine" Middleton was the quietest of Granddaddy's siblings. Her spirit was calming. Being in her presence was like sitting at the shores of an ocean. Her seemingly still demeanor often made me wonder what storms lie beneath. I knew only what I was told by older family members with slippery tongues. But I chose to believe what Pine told me about herself through no words at all. Her actions told her story.

Pine was the first and truest example of humility I had ever seen. She was a devoted wife whose ability to stick by her husband was known and admired by many on Liberty Hill. Aunt Pine often led a very intoxicated Uncle Jack out of the middle of Montague Avenue, in front of Granddaddy's house, back to their home. She was also a loving mother. Darryl and Cheryl were generational testaments of her kindness. They worked hard for the city of North Charleston. Aunt Pine was also a patient caregiver.

Aunt Pine took care of a young boy named Corey, who had autism. The few summer afternoons I spent at her house, when I was ten, were eye-opening. Corey never spoke but was attached to Aunt Pine by the hip. I knew Corey was not like my other cousins who I enjoyed playing with in Aunt Pine's yard. Every step he made seemed unsure. His only sure steps were towards her. Aunt Pine moved with ease as Corey followed. He clung to the security of their connection. Occasionally, she gently touched his head or shoulders. Corey knew, even while she was busy cleaning or cooking, Aunt Pine loved him.

I saw that same love and affection as she got to work in Granddaddy's kitchen. Aunt Pine did not ask any questions or say a word. She simply started to clean. Her skinny arms stretched deep into the cabinets to take every canned good and boxed item out for inspection. She wiped down the cabinets, making sure to reach every corner. After placing all the items back, she moved to the fridge and repeated the process. Moving at a steady pace, she threw away old food and disinfected surfaces. After the grunt work, the basics were next. The glasses on her face slid down her nose from the perspiration. She washed the dishes from breakfast and cleaned the sink. She wiped down the stove and finally, swept the floor. I watched her for hours. I offered to help but she insisted.

"No, it's ok. I got it."

There was something different about the help she provided that morning. It was a type of help I would rarely see again. She knew what needed to be done and she did what she could. Most apparent was the humble spirit with which Aunt Pine worked. She did not seek recognition or praise. The appreciation I so desperately wanted to give her seemed unnecessary to her.

"Aunt Pine. Thank you so much," I said, almost in tears. "I had no idea how I was going to get all of this done."

"It's alright," she replied.

I swear her face looked like an angel.

"You just have to take things one day at a time. Remember that, Quala."

"Yes ma'am." I wanted to hug her and be held by her spirit. But she left as quietly as she came. A fresh wave of energy overcame my body. I was ready for the parade of people to begin the next day.

A different person from Mama's outpatient treatment team was going to be in Granddaddy's house every weekday. I looked forward to meeting all the medical professionals who would be assisting with Mama's care. I was interested in learning their skill set. Most of all, I wanted to know how quickly they could get her well so we could go home.

A nurse came to the house just before noon on Tuesdays and Fridays and it was a different woman every week. Part of their duties was monitoring Mama's vitals and checking the feeding tube to make sure it was clean and working properly. The nurse also bathed Mama twice a week. I watched this process so I could take over once the visits stopped. I didn't realize the strength it took for Mama to get in and out of the bathtub. The nurse told me her weakness would not last long. She was right. Soon, the nurse only came once a week because Mama was strong enough to bathe alone.

The physical therapist came every week as well. Mama was still wearing a cast on her right leg. She could walk but needed some help when she got tired. This therapist focused on Mama's leg healing properly to regain her full range of motion. Using different exercises, the doctor showed her how to use the countertop to balance and stretch the limb. Mama enjoyed those leg lifts. The therapist also suggested taking advantage of Granddaddy's large yard. One of the three gardens in the backyard was encompassed by a dirt driveway. It was often used to get out of the yard when a number of people were at the house. The therapist instructed her to try walking a lap around the circle each day. Mama barely made it halfway around at first, but as time passed, she got stronger and quicker.

The speech therapist was an interesting man. Dr. Moss was a short, bald white man with glasses and a beard filled with gray hair. He explained his visits would depend on his teaching schedule at South Carolina State University. His drive to and from Orangeburg affected the time available for patients. Revealing that information went a long way with me. I thought he was a bit impersonal. It was clear he wasn't too keen on the idea of a teenager being a primary caregiver. Dr. Moss never spoke directly to me until I told him I was a college-bound, high school senior. His personality did not soften but he was willing to answer questions about the university. As he got to know me, he was much more open to working together.

Speech therapy was more memory therapy than anything else. It involved a lot of cognitive exercises and they reminded me of the $25,000 Pyramid game show. Dr. Moss wrote many different categories on index cards. He wanted her to practice the categories every day and list as many as possible. They ranged from colors to fruit and veggies to cities and states. He gave her a starting goal of five for each category with hopes of increasing each week. These exercises were difficult for Mama. Most days, she named about three of each. I was impatient. I felt pressured to improve her cognition by each week's session. I also used it as an indicator of her progress and how long it would be before we could go home. Dr. Moss explained it would take time for these skills to return. I tried to be patient, but I wanted my Mama back.

Another large part of Mama's outpatient treatment was occupational therapy which focused on her ability to do typical meaningful activities such as cooking, cleaning, and practicing other hobbies. The goal was to get her as close to her old routine as possible. I interpreted this as getting her as close to her old self as possible. The first session was assessing her current condition and painting a picture of Sandra Porterfield before the accident. Dr. Perry asked me a lot of questions about who she was and what she liked to do. I told him about her love of ceramics.

"See," I said, pointing at the beautiful, glossed statues sitting on the living room table. "She painted those for my grandmother. And our house is full of stuff she painted."

"What else did she enjoy?" Dr. Perry asked with sincere eyes.

"Mama was regularly active in our church. She taught Sunday School and loved the usher board."

Then he asked what kind of mother she was. The question made sense, but the answer was not so easy to understand. I talked about how present she was, attending every one of my competitions and events. Our relationship was not a part of my answer. I did not think those details were necessary especially since we were getting the fresh start we discussed before we left on my spring break.

Dr. Perry listened and took a lot of notes. The first thing he advised me of was the very slim chance Mama would ever drive again. Her reflexes were no longer quick enough to react to that kind of stimulus. The outlook was much more positive for basic activity. Dr. Perry could tell from talking to Mama, she was eager to get active. He suggested we start doing things around the house together. At the very least, encourage her to be in the room where activity was occurring, such as having her sit and watch Grandaddy, and I cook or tend to his gardens. Sessions started at twice a week for a while but were gradually reduced to once a week.

The social worker was the thread through all of Mama's outpatient care. I liked her. Giselle was much more of a pleasure to work with than anyone I met. She was kind, patient, listened to my concerns, and answered my questions. If she did not have an answer, she would make every effort to get it. Giselle also provided her contact information. While the others did the same, for her, the step did not seem procedural. It felt genuine.

The duration of outpatient care varied. The physical therapist estimated approximately six weeks. The plan was for Mama's cast to come off in three weeks and continue sessions through the summer for muscle strengthening. Speech and occupational therapy were a different story. Both estimated months of treatment and it all depended on her progress. I tried to look ahead towards August. It was going to be a full month with both Mama and my birthdays. August kicked off with my scholarship pageant, followed by the start of my senior year. Somehow, none of these upcoming events seemed as exciting as they did before Mama's accident. I couldn't see past this first week of June. The future was clouded with doctor appointments, treatment sessions, and hope that I could soon go home.

Facing Responsibility

The alarm was loud. The alarm was relentless. The alarm was unforgiving. And so was she.

"I'm going to tell them to turn the shit off!"

"There's nobody over there," I said. "I told you. Mr. McCant's has been closed since Hugo."

"Well, call the police!"

"That's what the alarm is for," I tried to explain. "To get somebody out here."

"Well, dammit! I'll call."

She tried to find the phone. Thankfully, it was out of sight and out of her reach.

"What are you going to say?" I asked, frustrated.

"I'm go'n tell them to come and cut the shit off. Then I'm go'n tell them to carry you and the McCants to jail!"

The loud, incessant noise of the alarm was a trigger for Mama. Old McCant's filling station was right next door to Granddaddy's house, on the corner of Montague and Mixon; right where the stoplight hung to signify the boundaries of Liberty Hill. The McCants were nice to Granddaddy over the decades. The white family often used the circle around his garden to test drive cars they fixed in the repair shop. Hurricane Hugo had damaged the structure severely which led to the business ultimately closing. I'm sure looters may have played a role as well. The building was vacant, but the alarm system still operated and was annoyingly sensitive. The loud, repetitive blasts went off at any time throughout the day. Usually, it was because an obnoxious motorcycle or a stray dog cut the corner too close to the door.

The rooms at the back of Granddaddy's house faced the filling station. I heard the alarms occasionally. The noise was annoying, but

I got used to it. Someone usually turned it off within ten to fifteen minutes. While the noise was an occasional nuisance for me, it was torture for Mama. Her old room was at the back of the house as well. The alarm had gone off several times since she returned from the hospital. Every false alarm led to a very real episode. The alarm went off. The dogs would start to bark, and she would explode into a fit of rage. I dreaded the alarm not only for the noise but because I knew what was coming.

The first episode was intense and extremely scary. I was sitting in a chair, watching TV while she and Granddaddy were resting in their bedrooms. The noise was always a bit frightening at first. About a minute had passed when she emerged from her bedroom. She limped down the hallway towards me, holding the walls to steady herself.

"What the fuck is that?" she yelled.

The noise startled her, and I tried to calm her down.

"It's just the alarm over at McCant's," I answered.

"Well go tell them to turn it off," she demanded.

I stared at her. I had to remind myself of her memory loss. Mama barely remembered her first wedding in the yard when she was 19. A detail like the business next door closing was lost. I tried to gently explain.

"I can't. Mr. McCant's is closed down. Remember?" Of course, she didn't. The words just came out by reflex but I held out hope. "Nobody's over there."

She limped a little closer. "Well, then you go turn it off!"

I was confused. "Huh?"

"Dammit. I said go cut the shit off!" She was louder and closer.

"I don't know what you want me to do," I pleaded.

"Bitch, you don't know who you messin' with." She heaved a weird chuckle. "You don't know. You don't know me."

I fearfully looked into her eyes. She was right. I didn't know her. This was not like the verbal beatings I received as a little girl. This

103

was very different. It felt different. This woman was not yelling at her daughter. She was threatening her enemy.

I stood and backed away towards Granddaddy's bedroom. His door was open to the living room.

"Granddaddy, please tell her I can't do anything about the alarm." I was in his doorway, hoping they could see each other.

"Sandra. Calm down. It'll stop in a few minutes. Just sit down. Rest your nerves," he yelled from his bed.

She stood in front of me for a second. The dogs stopped barking and she sat on the sofa. The alarm finally stopped. She did not respond to the silence. This woman watched television as if nothing happened. My face still felt the heat of her anger, along with the knots in the pit of my stomach. I was afraid to move and did not want to walk. A real fear paralyzed me from walking through the path between her view of the TV. If she saw me, it might trigger her rage again. But I could not stay in the room with her so I quickly walked to Cole's room.

I sat on the bed, still shaking. Thank God Granddaddy was home. Thinking about how it could have played out if I were alone with her, was almost too much. I tried to process what had just happened. That was not my Mama. Where was my Mama? The woman sitting in the living room did not respond to reason. My frustration angered her. My fear empowered her. And only my grandfather's voice calmed her. I had felt the wrath of my Mama. Bruised skin, a bloody nose, and a lot of hurt feelings were evidence. Through it all, I never questioned her love for me. I never feared for my life. This woman made me do both.

Various episodes occurred throughout the summer. Triggers were sometimes unpredictable. The merciless heat and humidity did not help matters. Cooling off in Granddaddy's house was like trying to find water in a desert. A large fan at the front of the house did a decent job keeping the living area cool. God help you if you stepped out of its range. We kept the kitchen door closed to prevent the house from feeling like we were being baked in every room. Still, my body felt like a broiling T-bone. I was grateful for the large trees in the backyard cascading over the back of the house. They provided a nice shade when I wanted to retreat to Cole's room.

We went to visit Cole soon after he was transferred from the county jail. Approved visitors were on a list and were only allowed to come on Saturdays. Dress code restrictions did not allow us to wear denim due to the inmate uniforms. They wore denim jeans and a shirt with their number on it. I liked the uniforms. I conveniently disregarded the purpose of the prison garb and saw something trendy about them. They appealed to me so much; I asked Cole if he could have one sent to me for my birthday. He got a kick out of the idea and tried to grant my request. I was excited to be able to wear something I knew no one at school would have. The reason for my excitement was also the reason the prison did not allow him to send one to me. A prison uniform is not a style or badge of honor. He sent me a handmade Barney birthday card instead.

Visiting Cole was not like visiting Mama at the mental facility after her nervous breakdown. That place was like a freaking retreat compared to Cole's new residence. The ride was shorter to see him but getting in was much more tedious. We drove 45 minutes to the prison. A long line greeted us when we arrived for our visit. The first checkpoint was where the visitor dress code was strictly enforced. Several females were turned away at the gate because of violations from wearing jeans to outfits that were too revealing. A table sat outside where we presented our IDs and gave the name of the inmate we came to see. If we passed that inspection, we were allowed through the first door into a corridor. The doors locked in front of and behind us. Guards checked our IDs again. We waited to pass through metal detectors before being escorted to the visiting room where we waited for Cole.

The visiting room looked like a large cafeteria at a poorly funded school. The room was filled with square tables and hard chairs. A few vending machines lined the walls along with the prison guards. Harsh fluorescent tube lights lit the room. The walls were painted a light, simple crème color. Loud bells indicated when an inmate was being escorted into the room.

During the first visit, I sat at a table with Granddaddy and my mother who hardly spoke. She was fresh out of the hospital with the tube still attached to her stomach. I was surprised the guard let her through. Cole asked to see it. He was thrown at the sight when I discreetly lifted her shirt. She was unfazed.

Granddaddy was a little more talkative. He asked a lot of questions, mostly out of concern. Cole and I spoke on the phone but seeing him was more comforting, though it was strange. My brother looked the same. He acted the same. Nothing was different about who Cole was. I was not sure if this was a good thing or a bad thing. Maybe, he was doing what the other inmates in the room seemed to be doing, making the best of a bad situation. I wanted more. I wanted Cole to show remorse for what Granddaddy was going through because of him. My brother owed him an apology for his actions. And he owed me an apology for making me go through this alone.

The responsibility of two households was on my shoulders. I had Mama's checkbook from when we retrieved her belongings from the car in Georgia. A key to the post office box she rented was among the items. I was able to see her bank statements and understand where she was financially. It did not permit me to go crazy at the mall. Utilities at Mama's house needed to be paid. Then, the hospital bills started coming. Mama's Medicaid covered many of the medical bills, but a few balances were remaining along with her prescriptions.

Mama received a monthly disability check due to her mental illness after an incident while she worked for Amtrak. I never knew what happened, only that Mama would never be employed again. She also received two monthly child support checks from my father which totaled $300. My name was on those checks too. I was able to deposit them and get a little cash when I showed identification. The bank was quite familiar with Mama and Granddaddy. I discovered his name was on her account as well. These two were connected in every freaking way.

Budgeting came pretty easy to me. Though she did not receive much income, Mama's expenses were minimal. I built a plan of attack on her hospital bills. Granddaddy's den became my little office, and I used an old notebook to keep track of Mama's finances. There was no desk in the room, but no one went in there except me. I sat on the small couch and laid out all the bills: prioritizing every expense, figuring out monthly payments that fit her income, and enabling her to pay off the hospital bills in twelve to eighteen months.

A little room was left for my expenses like gas money to drive around. There was money to buy the snacks I liked for Granddaddy's house. I also wanted to keep a small food supply at Mama's house since I still went there throughout the week. Going to Mama for money was no longer an option. The idea of asking Granddaddy for much of anything was daunting. I did not know how to explain that a jar of Snapple or a shower at Mama's house gave me the break I so desperately needed.

Then there was the upcoming school year. Senior year was expensive. I knew in a few months I would have to buy school clothes, pay senior dues, and get graduation attire. College application fees were looming. I did not let go of my dreams to attend a large university. It was my ticket off Liberty Hill. Going to a school in South Carolina was still out of the question. North Carolina, Georgia, and California were most appealing after a year of research. California was a long shot, but I liked fantasizing about going to UCLA for acting. UNC Charlotte was still on the table since I visited the campus. There were plans to visit several other universities before Mama's accident. I held on to the false hope of making the trips with Mama for a little while until her condition made it abundantly clear it was not going to happen. Ideas ran through my mind of making the trips alone. The idea was appealing at first but later led to a painful reality. I was managing Mama's money, taking care of her house, and taking care of her. There was no one to take care of me. I had to take care of myself.

Taking care of myself meant navigating the college application process alone. I had to figure out how to pay for my education. Mama's low income gave me access to financial aid, but I would need a whole lot more to make up the difference for the type of school I wanted to attend. Scholarships were a necessity. I spent a lot of time in the library during the last few weeks of my junior year. Large catalogs of college scholarships and grants covered the hard, wood tables where I sat. Most had specific requirements I could not meet. Parents had to have certain occupations or live in a certain area. Volunteering in a remote country might get me a couple thousand dollars. The only realistic way for me to get the kind of money I needed was to work with what I knew best.

I watched beauty pageants on television for as long as I can remember. The names of every black Miss America, Miss USA, and Miss Universe were etched in my memory with historical figures. Mama let me enter a small pageant the year before the accident. It was a nice introduction to competing on this stage. I hated the false beauty expectations, like makeup and lashes, but I enjoyed walking with confidence and performing. Talent and Interview were where I would soar past the competition. I used the first pageant and Miss North Charleston High for practice. Miss WPAL would be the next level with higher stakes.

WPAL was the oldest black radio station in Charleston. They had recently expanded to FM as well as their familiar AM dial. Every year the station sponsored a scholarship pageant for rising high school seniors in the tri-county area. My church youth advisor, Raquel, introduced me to the event years earlier. She and her best friend Jon took me to see it. They opened a new world for me.

Wearing a crown and a sash was my dream the moment I saw Debbye Turner crowned Miss America 1990. When Raquel and Jon took me to the Miss WPAL pageant, the dream seemed possible. I signed up for the contest as soon as I was eligible.

The initial meeting was before Mama's accident. She drove me to the radio station after school. I was super excited. Mama was excited for me too. I talked about the pageant constantly over the last two years. She knew this was something I wanted to do. I went inside for the meeting while Mama ran an errand. At the end of the meeting, I chatted with a few contestants. Full preparations would not begin for a few months. I told Mama all the information when I got in the car. We talked about the things I needed and planned to begin preparations after we returned from Spring Break. Since plans changed, I figured I would have to prepare alone. Thankfully, I was wrong.

Raquel was like a guardian angel over my soul since the night Mama didn't come home. She came to see me compete for Miss North Charleston High. The support of her presence was something I did not know I needed. Soon after, she and John were my coaches for the Miss WPAL pageant. They took me shopping for the casual wear competition. I met with Jon to show him the dance and monologue I put together for talent. As a trained performer, he was able to take what I came up with to another level with points of emphasis and upgraded choreography. He created a spectacular African outfit to match the music and theme of my monologue. He also designed a beautiful red gown for the evening wear competition. Jon and Raquel worked with me on walking with graceful confidence. They invested time and money and asked for nothing in return except that I do my best.

I committed to giving my all, starting from the first pageant rehearsal. Every Saturday morning, I drove downtown to practice the opening number with the other girls. This was another welcomed escape from everything happening at my grandfather's house. I didn't have to think about medications and appointments and therapy sessions. For a few hours, I was just the teenage girl I was supposed to be before the accident. I was the star Prince sang about in our opening number song. Every time we said, "Baby I'm a Star," I believed it.

After a very trying summer, the day finally came for me to shine. I invited a lot of good friends. Raquel and Jon were there. I wanted Willie to come but I had not seen him much since the beginning of the summer. He never felt truly welcome at Granddaddy's house. My biological father also crossed my mind. Daddy did not reach out after Mama's accident. I wondered if he knew how severe her injuries were. My biggest question was if he wondered who was taking care of me. Since the child support checks kept coming every month, I figured he either assumed things were okay or he didn't care. I told Granddaddy about the pageant. He did not ask questions about it. My grandfather seemed so uninterested; I wondered if he would even come. Getting Mama there was also a concern. I hoped by seeing me compete again, something would switch on in her memory to remind her she had a daughter. I invited Aunt Barbara who said she would bring Mama and Granddaddy if he was up to it.

Backstage, I did not think about who was in the audience. I was focused on the task at hand. Once we completed the opening number, I went into competitive mode. The stage turned into an imaginary runway where I strutted in my white, two-piece casual suit. Nerves dissipated during the dance and monologue, which went better than I expected. The costume Jon designed flowed beautifully with every move and every word. His creation for my evening wear was also flawless. I felt like a star on the red carpet as I floated across the stage in my red, off-the-shoulder, fishtail dress. Then it was time for the interview competition.

All the contestants stood on stage, waiting for our turn. This was the first chance for me to see who was in the audience. I scanned the faces. Raquel and Jon's loud cheers rang out every time I appeared.

K'Lani and her sister were there to support me too. Mama's face was visible right before my name was called for the final question. I lucked out. The question was one K'Lani practiced with me, a few weeks earlier. The answer still repeated in my head. Then, something happened. Doubts whispered loud enough to drown out the rehearsed response and my new answer did not sound intelligent enough. I questioned the maturity of my opinion on a local controversy. All summer, I was forced to grow up quickly. Thinking practically was more important than being allowed to dream. So, I gave a practical answer. I was articulate. I was intelligent. I expressed the opinion of an experienced adult. I expressed an opinion that was not my own. A forced smile curved my mouth as I turned. My heart sank. I knew I lost as soon as I walked away from the microphone.

First Runner-up was a good consolation prize. The sash came with a very tall, gold and faux wood trophy. Most importantly, I won $2000 in scholarship money. I was $2000 closer to getting past the railroad tracks. All the contestants took pictures after the pageant. I was proud of my performance overall. The same pride shined in the wide grins of Jon, Raquel, and all of my friends as they gathered around the stage to congratulate me. I could not say the same for one person.

Aunt Barbara managed to bring Mama to the pageant. She had on a familiar suit I loved. It seemed a little too big for her. They came to the stage afterward. There were no words of congratulations from her. She said nothing at all. Her face was void of pride or any other emotion. She barely looked at me.

"Raquel and Jon thought we could go eat together," I said.

"I'm ready to go home." She finally spoke.

"Yeah," Aunt Barbara replied. "I'm just gonna go ahead and get her home."

"Oh," I said. "OK, then."

At first, her face seemed blank. She seemed annoyed, rolling her eyes. I did not recognize this woman. She had on my Mama's clothes and my Mama's face. Her eyes were open, but they were cold and distant. I realized then, she was gone. My mama died in that car accident, and she was not coming back. All my hope followed Aunt Barbara and my mother as they walked out of the theater.

The Saturday Murder

I killed them. I killed my granddaddy's dogs.

As a child, I loved Little and Charaka. They were one of the reasons I enjoyed sleepovers at my grandparents' house. I liked feeding them and petting them. They were my playmates when I was alone. Sometimes, I got a bit rambunctious using Little as my dance partner to impress imaginary Star Search judges. She would put up with it for a few minutes before cueing the end of the dance with a growl or a snap at my fingers. One bite was enough to make me go solo.

Weekend sleepovers made taking care of the dogs a fun project when I was a kid but living with them was very different. Since moving in with Granddaddy after the accident, daily contact meant being exposed to the consequences of their lack of proper grooming. By mid-June, I found myself frantically scratching my legs while sitting in the living room. My eyes nearly popped out of my head, the first time I saw the tiny, dark creature on my skin. As I went to flick it off me, the thing jumped from one spot on my leg to another and then onto the carpet.

"Oh my God," I shouted!

My body was a playground for fleas. The problem got worse as summer's humid heat intensified. I told Granddaddy about the infestation. He gave me money to buy the dogs' flea collars. This helped Little and Charaka a bit but the fleas had already found new homes in the carpet and on me. I did not understand. No one else seemed bothered by the invaders. What was it about me that attracted them? I felt like an animal was constantly attacking my body. Every day I was scratching. I would scan my legs and arms for the tiny hopping critters. I was paranoid about seeing or feeling one on me.

There were nights I didn't sleep for fear of the fleas crawling over my body or worse.

Living in Granddaddy's house was miserable as the Fourth of July approached. The room I slept in was not mine. A stranger was walking around with my Mama's body. I was fending off fleas and scratching myself raw. The summer before my senior year had turned into a physical and emotional fight to keep my sanity. Oftentimes, the only way to survive was to retreat. I usually tried to get away on Saturday evenings.

It was easy to forget I was a teenager after a week of cooking, cleaning, observing therapy sessions, giving medication, and helping with exercises. I tried to remind myself by going to my Aunt Debbie's house or visiting my friend, Mosheera, at work. Aunt Debbie was Granddaddy's youngest daughter. She was short, spunky, and physically active. Aunt Debbie walked to her job every weekday morning at six and coached community tee-ball in the afternoons. Her oldest daughter, Chanel, was one of my favorite cousins. We were only two years apart, but I admired her confidence and outspoken personality. Mosheera was an old friend from the Buist days. We reconnected as students at North Charleston High. She was funny and a joy to be around. On Saturdays when I found an escape, I made sure everything was done at Granddaddy's by six o'clock in the evening. Then, I would head out to the fast-food place where Mosheera worked, or to Aunt Debbie's.

The last Saturday in June, I was alone with my mother and the dogs the entire afternoon. Luckily, Willie showed up for what would be his last time at Granddaddy's house. He knew I was struggling. I asked if he could stay while I went somewhere. Anywhere. Thankfully, he said yes. I walked outside and looked at Mama's car just sitting there. It looked as if it was dying like the old brown Dodge sitting across from it. That car had been settling in the dirt since before Grandmama died. It was partly used for extra storage of junk Granddaddy did not care about. The idea of Mama's car being discarded as junk pissed me off. I was not going to let him do that to her stuff. I would not let him do that to me. So, I took Mama's Buick instead of the Chrysler.

I just wanted to feel some sense of the life I was supposed to have. Granddaddy was not coming back until later that evening, so he would never know. I drove to Chanel's house. We laughed loudly and played with her little sisters. The car, Granddaddy's house, and the woman with Mama's face were purposefully placed in the back of my mind until Aunt Debbie came to her daughter's bedroom.

"Quala. You know the tags expire on your car at the end of the month?"

I had no idea what she was talking about. I just told her I would take care of it. The hours were going by fast when I glanced at my watch. Getting back before Granddaddy was crucial. I said good night to everyone and quickly got in the car.

My heart sank when I pulled into the driveway and saw the big red truck. I went straight back to the bedroom where Willie was sitting at my mother's bedside. He told me Granddaddy was not angry, but I needed to apologize. I slowly walked to his bedroom. He was lying on the bed, staring at nothing. The room was dimly lit with the one nightstand lamp illuminating his face. I stepped in through the living room.

"Granddaddy?" He looked at me. "I'm sorry for taking Mama's car. I should have asked you. I thought it would be ok since the tags don't expire until next month."

He looked blankly at me. I could tell he knew I was dishing out crap. "Yeah, but there's no insurance on that car anymore," he said. "There was no need to renew it."

"Oh." My heart sank. Looking at him, I was torn. No need to renew it? What about me? What about Mama? Did he know she was never coming back? He just gave up, so I had to give up too? I hated how pieces of the life I knew were being taken from me. I also hated

Granddaddy's disappointment in me which I had never experienced. My defiance surprised him, and my actions hurt him.

Independence Day came with no real celebration. Driving Mama's car was no longer an option, but I continued my weekend escapes. Getting out of the house was particularly hard one Saturday towards the end of July. There was nothing memorable about the day except the usual summer heat. Finishing up my duties seemed to take longer. The more time it took to get things done, the more inadequate I felt. Dinner was not to my grandfather's liking. My mother had an episode of rage earlier in the afternoon. Topping it off, I was still fighting those dern fleas! I sprayed the carpet with flea repellant but it was not working. I was still scratching and growing more anxious as the hours passed. My mind could not settle. The walls were closing in on me.

Finally, a little before six o'clock, the house calmed down. Granddaddy lay in his bedroom while my mother sat on the living room sofa, watching television. I walked out the door, desperate for peace, normalcy, and sanity. My desperation did not dissipate this gnawing feeling that I should not go. I stepped off the back porch, trying to silence the voice telling me not to leave.

It's not that bad. The voice whispered on my skin. *It's not that serious. You don't have to get away.* I kept walking through the yard. *You're just saying it's bad so you can leave. You just want to hang out with your friends.*

"Why is that so bad?!" I snapped. "Can't I have some fun? Even if it's just standing around at Wendy's? I'm sixteen!"

I saw the white 1984 Chrysler LeBaron Granddaddy made me drive. Mama's Buick was parked in the yard to the left. Every time I looked at the two cars, my heart pounded in anger. The fact of not being able to drive my Mama's car was a reminder of how she was snatched from me along with life as I knew it.

"I'm going," I said as I walked towards the LeBaron. I silenced the voice.

Little and Charaka always followed me around outside when I was leaving. I saw them as I approached the car. I opened the door and got in. I sat on the red cushioned seat with one foot on the mat and the other still outside. Little and Charaka stood in the door opening. They were looking at me with eyes attempting to speak. I looked back at them. I always thought they were the prettiest Chihuahuas on the planet. Little was the smaller one. She was tri-colored with a black body, brown tipped ears with a brown triangle patch on her head pointing between her eyes, and a white-tipped tail. Her son, Charaka, was also black with browning gray patches all over. Their eyes were round and dark but happy. They usually made me happy too but not this Saturday evening. Looking into their eyes, I felt guilty. The voice I thought was silenced, had taken shape. It was alive and staring at me through Little's eyes. Suddenly, I was afraid. The vision of the worst scenario flashed on the screen of my mind. But it wouldn't happen for real, right? No. It couldn't happen.

"I have to go. Y'all need to move," I told them.

I put my leg inside. I swear, it looked like they smiled at me as they backed away and I closed the door. I turned the key in the ignition. I sat there for a second. Did they move? They usually did. I put the car in reverse. They always backed away from moving vehicles in the yard. I slowly pressed the gas. The muffled yelp told me one of them had not backed away this time. I stopped immediately.

"Please, God. Please, God," I said, hoping against what I knew to be true.

I opened the door to the gruesome reality. Charaka stood there, helplessly watching his mother's torso under the tire, her legs desperately kicking, running for the life I was taking from her. I screamed in horror. I jumped back in the car quickly trying to think of how to save her. I put the car in reverse and pressed the gas. I don't know how far I went before breaking and putting the car in park. I opened the door. I did not look down as I got out, for fear I would see the truth, but Charaka was still in my view. He was in the same spot with the same helpless look on his face.

I ran into the house. In a matter of seconds, I had to figure out how to tell Granddaddy I had done the worst thing I could do. I was shaking when I got to his room.

"Granddaddy, something's wrong with Little."

He was laying down on his bed. "What? What's wrong with her?"

"I hit her. Oh, God. I hit her. I'm so sorry."

He got up without saying a word. He put on his shoes and went outside. I could not move, hoping against all odds she would survive. Knowing I may have killed her was almost unbearable. After a few minutes, my grandfather returned. I saw him looking for something. I had to ask.

"Is she…?" I couldn't finish.

"No, she's gone," he said, confirming my fear.

I was frozen. Granddaddy gathered a few supplies as I stood, still frozen, watching him through his open bedroom door. Then he went back out.

Disbelief stunned my body. I looked to the left, out of his other doorway that led to the living room. The green, flea sprayed carpet was more vivid. My mother stared at the television, completely oblivious to what was happening. I could not run to my Mama for solace. Thoughts about what Granddaddy was having to do outside crept into my head. They made my limbs tremble. Where was Willie? I needed him. I needed someone. There was no comfort. There was no sense of home in this house.

The screen door opened and slammed. Granddaddy was back. His quiet sadness scared me. I felt his hurt as he walked in from burying his beloved dog in the far, back, corner of the big garden. I wondered if he hated me. The pain I caused him was too great. I needed to go. It felt wrong to ask. Respect was all I could give and it only came with permission. I looked at Granddaddy. While I tried my best to explain, he stopped me and simply said, "Go ahead."

I hesitated. Maybe he didn't want me there either. I turned and went out the door.

I was numb, walking towards the car. Then fear overtook my senses when I came around to the driver's side. Charaka was still there. He was in the same spot I left him, staring. Hadn't he followed Granddaddy to say goodbye to his mother? The image of him watching her being carried away was becoming clear. He looked up at me trying to get the image out of my head. I froze. His eyes were darker than usual. He did not move. Neither did I. I was so afraid. Then, without growling, he slowly stepped toward me. That was enough to make me take off running. I prayed he was not behind me when I ran into the house.

"Granddaddy! Granddaddy!" I went straight to his bedroom. "I'm so sorry. But can you please get Charaka?"

"What?" Granddaddy said, looking at me, confused.

"I went to get in the car and he...I just..." I was shaking. "Just, please. Can you get him?"

He smiled as he sat upon the bed. "Ok. I'll get him."

He put his shoes back on and went outside. Minutes passed before I heard the screen door slam again when he returned.

"Alright. He's in the utility room," he said, sitting down on his bed.

"Thank you. Granddaddy, I'm sorry. I'm so sorry."
He looked at me.

"It was an accident, Quala. You can't help accidents. Just go ahead."

He needed me out of his face. I quickly left and headed to my cousin's house. Fear and guilt gripped my chest while I was there. I had to call Granddaddy to ask him to make sure Charaka was still secured before I came back that evening.

The next several days were eerie. Charaka began to follow me everywhere. He sat at my feet in the living room when I watched TV. He followed me up and down the hall. He would be at Cole's door when I opened it in the mornings. He tried to come into the bedroom in the evenings. All the while, Charaka never growled at me. He just looked at me with a strange, sad smile on his face. I started to be okay with his presence. If following me around, somehow brought him some comfort, who was I to take it away from him? Maybe this was part of my restitution for taking his mother. As the days passed, my fear subsided. I started to see what I hoped was forgiveness in his eyes. Though, I never forgave myself.

One afternoon, I noticed Charaka was not following me around. I realized I had not seen him all day. I thought his grieving was over. The next day, I returned from an errand and saw him on Granddaddy's large back porch. I was so relieved. He had found a little space on the corner amongst the plants. There, he slept. The following day, I saw him there again. I knew something was off but I was too afraid and ashamed to say anything. Then one day, he wasn't there.

"You noticed you haven't seen Charaka?" Granddaddy asked.

"No, I noticed. But I saw him sleeping on the porch the day before yesterday."

He shook his head. "He wasn't sleeping."

The guilt came rushing back. "No," I cried.

"I found him yesterday. I buried him in the yard with Little."

I could not respond. I wanted to turn back time. I wanted to give Granddaddy his dogs back. I wanted to give him his house back. I wanted my Mama. I wanted my life back. But the summer had painfully taught me that it was not possible. The dogs were gone. Mama was gone. Summer was over…and my mourning season began.

A Way Out

Praying was a tradition my family counted on. Growing up, they swore it changed things, but I had yet to see any real differences myself. I thought about my days at Buist Academy. I asked Him to stop the bullying, but he didn't. It continued right up to the night of commencement. I thought about the choir director. I asked after the first time, to never let it happen again. It did happen…again and again. I asked him to soften Mama so she would stop beating and belittling me. As soon as things were about to change between us, He took her away.

When Mama's accident happened, it brought me back to my knees. I would be in Cole's room with the door closed, pleading with him to make it better. I asked him to heal her and bring Mama back. I got nothing. A few times after getting off my knees, my mother would have a horrible episode. I opened the bedroom door when she was just about to turn the knob. A grimace covered her face as she lunged at my arm and cursed at me about a noise or something else bothering her. They were violent confirmations that my prayers were pointless.

But I kept going back to Him. I didn't know what else to do. After the Miss WPAL pageant, I collapsed on Cole's bed. I didn't have the strength to get on my knees.

"Say something!" I exclaimed, curled up on the bed.

I had no idea what to listen for. Clichés or colloquialisms were not enough. People at church often spewed overused Bible verses. They all said the same thing.

"Hang in there. You know all things work together for good."
I wanted to strangle the vocal cords of every person who said it. Their words of comfort seemed disingenuous. People seemed to be more curious than concerned. The fact that the curious ones used

121

God's words angered me to my soul. Hearing directly from Him became vital to my sanity.

"I need you to say something," I said, late that night.
I waited to hear His voice. Rolling thunder or some deep celestial tone was not necessary. Love was what I needed to hear; words to comfort me and ease my pain. I desperately searched through his words until finally, He spoke. In Bible pages, through the silence, He spoke.

"I'm here. I've always been here." He said through Isaiah.

"Yeah right," I retorted.

"We got together when you were so very young. You were sad and abandoned."

"You left me," I snapped.

"For a moment, I left you."

"A moment?! It's been years!"

"For me, a thousand years are like one day."

"Well, that's great. I'm never getting out of this hell," I said, hopelessly.

"No, I swear to you. This will not last forever. I will get you out of this. I promise you. I will not leave you. Your dreams matter to me. You matter to me."

I listened to His promises. He talked about my future and our relationship. It was comforting but hard to believe. The reality I was living, blocked the view of this future He spoke of. His words were nice to hear but they were not easing my pain. They were making me bitter. I wanted to walk away. I wanted to let go of the whole idea of His very existence. But something kept pulling me back in. He just would not let me go.

The first day of my senior year was the day after I turned 17. The crew gave me a personalized birthday card after school. It was the only acknowledgment of my birthday besides Cole's phone call from prison. Many milestones passed unnoticed. Taking senior pictures, buying my cap and gown, and Homecoming was more like momentary distractions instead of memories to be made. I wanted to be excited. I wanted to be happy. Each day I tried to walk the halls with the same smile I wore the last three years, but it grew more difficult as the school year progressed. Nothing was the same.

Afternoons usually spent preparing for band competitions were spent preparing meals. I think Granddaddy hated my cooking. What I did never seemed up to his standards. His silence at my meals screamed dissatisfaction. I did not have the seasoned skills of Grandmama or his sister, Aunty Mina, but I tried hard. Unfortunately, basic dishes were all Mama taught me before the accident. As Thanksgiving quickly approached, my lack of ability made the idea of cooking a holiday meal quite daunting. I was not looking forward to it.

Sitting alone at the dining room table, I was trying to figure out what to do when I heard a knock at the door. I scoffed as I went to answer. It was around eleven o'clock in the morning. Holiday visitors were expected but I didn't think they would start this early. My mouth nearly hit the floor when I opened Granddaddy's back door. The ladies came in like Wonder Women on Thanksgiving morning. I recognized the first face. She was a member of Abundant Life and my friend's mother. One of Mama's fellow usher board members was behind her. A few other church ladies followed into the kitchen with tin pans filled with a turkey and all the fixings.

"Happy Thanksgiving," they said, one after the other, as they entered.

They went about placing the pans on the kitchen table and counters. They placed the turkey in the oven and gave me reheating instructions. One of the ladies went out again and returned with bottles of soda and tea. It was amazing. They saved Thanksgiving and left as quickly as they came.

Granddaddy was touched by the generosity of my church. I think he was also relieved. He knew I was trying to plan dinner. I wanted to show him I was able to take care of a house. The Wonder Women of Abundant Life saved his day as much as they saved mine. Later, he and my mother sat at the dining room table as I fixed plates for each of us. He said the blessing and we dug in. I thought about Cole. I wondered what it was like to spend Thanksgiving in prison. He called and seemed okay. Still, I knew it had to be hard for him.

The house returned to its gloomy atmosphere when we finished eating. Granddaddy went to his room. My mother, Sandra, sat on the sofa just outside his door and watched TV. I cleared the table and cleaned the kitchen. My anxiety was gone but the sadness still loomed over me.

I discovered many ways to come from under the sadness. School was always a weird place of retreat. I forgot it was meant to be a place of education and it was very evident in my grades. There were no consequences for my subpar academic performance. No one questioned how I was doing in school. No one asked to see my report cards. I simply signed Mama's name myself. My focus was passing the three classes I knew were necessary for me to graduate. I rarely showed up for the other two. The sporadic attendance to Pre-Calculus finally caught the attention of the senior class vice principal. Since I had a good reputation with school administration and a clean record up to that point, I was able to sweet-talk the class off my schedule. I failed the other class.

Failure was not an option for Honors English. I attended regularly but wasn't completing assignments. Those that were completed barely met the minimum criteria. My teacher knew this was not typical for me. Mrs. Pavlisko was also my tenth-grade English teacher. She had seen my award-winning speeches and received thorough reports from me in the past. She read outstanding poetry and essays I had written. Mrs. Pavlisko was looking forward to my work as a senior and was surprised when I began turning in work below my potential. She was shocked when she had to give me detention for disrupting class. I sat numbly in her classroom, after school. The blonde, short-haired teacher looked at me from her desk, puzzled.

"What is going on with you, Ruthenna?" she asked, "This is not like you at all."

If you only knew, I thought. This woman could not fathom what was happening in my life.

"I know your Mom is sick. How's she doing?"
I felt the tears coming and fought them back. I was not going to cry in front of this woman.

"She's getting better," I replied. "She still doesn't remember me."

"She doesn't remember you?"

"No."

Mrs. Pavlisko was confused. She had no idea of the extent of my mother's condition. I continued, "She probably won't ever get her full memory back."

"I'm so sorry, Ruthenna. She's home now, right?"

"Well, we moved in with my grandfather so I can take care of them both in the same place."

She was quiet. I saw the pity in her eyes and felt her concern. She was visibly uncomfortable, shifting in her seat. Her questions went past a point she was not prepared to cross. I decided to lead her back.

"Actually, I was thinking of taking her to that play you said we could see for extra credit. I think it would be a nice outing for her." She followed my lead.

"Yes, it probably will. Let me know if you go."
The bell rang signaling the end of detention. She was relieved to dismiss me.

I drove home, as I often did after school. Mama's house was another retreat for me. Showers were like an oasis there. The fridge and the cupboards were stocked with my favorite snacks I bought. I listened to cassette tapes on my stereo. At first, being in my bedroom or sitting in the den was nice. It was familiar and comforting. Over time, however, the silence grew into a reminder of what I lost. There were days I sat on the floor with the shades pulled. I constantly allowed my mind to wonder where I would be if the accident had not happened and how my life would be different or better. My mind turned to how the accident might have been prevented. I wanted my own car so badly. I wanted independence. Mama was excited to be able to give it to me.

Sitting on the floor in the darkness, I saw the mangled, red, two-door hatchback in the Georgia junkyard. I saw some of Mama's teeth wrapped in a napkin, in a zip-loc bag Aunt Barbara gave me. I tried to rub the memories from my eyes and out of my mind. The memories only changed to visions of Little and Charaka. The images flooded my body with guilt and regret. At only seventeen years old, I managed to take three souls from this world in less than six months.

Guilt ravaged my body. If alcohol fixed bruises on the outside, maybe it dulled pain on the inside. I figured since it worked for Willie, he would be willing to provide what I needed. My Stepdaddy realized I was spending afternoons at home when he walked by one day. He came to the door when he saw the Chrysler LeBaron in the driveway. He never questioned why I was there alone. We talked for a little while before I asked him to buy some wine coolers for me. He was reluctant at first. I told him I just liked the taste of it.

"You always say it's basically just Kool-Aid anyway," I said, trying to convince him.
I knew hitting him with his own words would get me what I wanted. He agreed to buy them but only once.

The six-pack did not last long. It wasn't strong enough either. There was no way I could ask Willie for more. Then I remembered all the bottles of liquor in Cole's room. So, at night I took sips when I knew my mother and Grandfather were asleep. Sometimes I mixed portions of Crown Royal with Welch's grape soda like I saw Willie do many times. There was a tasty kick to the drink which made it seem harmless. The homemade cocktail became a nightly routine. I always tried to be careful not to drink too much. Eventually, the drinks ran out and the images returned.

Christmas came and went. A church conference in Baltimore, Maryland provided a much-needed distraction. Granddaddy's health was slowly improving. My mother only had occupational therapy which was suspended for the holiday. Aunt Barbara agreed to check on them daily while I was away. Those four days were a welcomed break. I still found myself thinking about what was waiting for me when I returned. I worried if leaving was selfish or irresponsible. The conference was something I would have done if the accident did not happen. I would have felt robbed if I did not go. The battle in my head made the trip almost pointless. I came back on New Year's Eve feeling worse than before I left.

The second semester of my senior year began on a very poor academic note. We were given all of Christmas break and the first week to work on a major Teacher Cadet project. The class was made up of select students with high academic achievement and leadership skills to steer them towards a teaching career. I loved the class mostly for the creative style of Mrs. Lavely. She was also my drama teacher as a freshman. I wanted to impress her with my work. The project required us to design our own preschool classroom based on what we learned about child psychology and education since the start of the school year. This assignment was exciting. I loved the idea of creating my own space. The problem was I felt like I had no space to call my own.

I never did schoolwork at Granddaddy's house. It felt wrong somehow. This project required a sizable, unobstructed area to work. Mama's house had space along with the necessary, uninterrupted time. What I did not have were uninterrupted thoughts. My mind was constantly distracted by my reality. An idea for a play section with vibrant colors would come to my head. Then it would be erased by the image of my mother staring at me with lifeless eyes. I would see alphabet letters stacked in the corner of a room but with one violent swoop, they were knocked over by my mother's hand. For days, I sat in my bedroom and stared at the blank poster board. Sometimes I sketched something and erase it. Buying more poster boards led to failed attempts at starting over. As the due date quickly approached, I felt overwhelmed. After a while, apathy set in. No one cared about my grades. So, why should I? I didn't need the class to graduate anyway. Finally, I just gave up.

Monday morning, I sat at my desk as everyone presented their projects. Mrs. Lavely spread the presentations over multiple days. It seemed like she was trying to give me extra time to turn in my project. Throwing something together crossed my mind but I just could not submit trashy work. Part of me wanted Mrs. Lavely to ask why I was not turning in my assignments. She never did but I still felt her disappointment. I just didn't care.

There was something liberating about apathy. The battle to hold on to sanity or to the future I always wanted was exhausting. I was tired of fighting. Every day felt like the battle was getting worse and I was tired of fighting alone. I spent more hours sitting on the floor of my room in darkness. It was nice not having something over my head when I decided to give up on the project. I wondered if giving up completely would work for everything in my head too.

Giving up was a constant thought since last summer. The idea started as fleeting. I asked myself what would happen if I did it. Most of the time, I was too afraid of the unknown to seriously consider it. With apathy setting in, the fear was dissipating. I considered different methods. A young girl from church hung herself but that sounded too painful. The revolver Mama used to shoot my father was still in a leather case in her bedroom. The irony of using the same gun made me laugh a little. It almost seemed vengeful. I wanted my family to feel the pain of my death. Aunt Barbara needed to face responsibility for disregarding my pain. Cousins should hurt for ignoring my struggle. I was already a footnote in their eyes. Non-existence was the next logical step. This was my hope but I knew it was false hope. My family would mourn for a little while with typical traditions and conversations about how they didn't know. Then they would move on with their lives with occasional stories where my name might pop up.

Their possible apathy did not affect mine. One afternoon, I went searching for the leather case. While searching, the memory of my Aunt Dorothy crossed my mind. She was my favorite aunt when I was a little girl. I remembered getting the news when she passed away.

"She died in her sleep," Grandmama replied when I asked how. It seemed so peaceful and natural. I liked the idea of just drifting away. There was a pill bottle in the bathroom. I stopped searching for the case. This method seemed more like my own. Besides, doing what my Buist classmate did felt like I would be taking something away from her.

I thought about Leah often. A romanticized image of her death was branded on my brain. I saw it as I opened the medicine cabinet. All of Leah's senses were probably stimulated. She saw the ocean. She heard the music. She smelled the waves. She felt the breeze. I took down the pill bottle. I poured the pills in my hand and began to take one and then two. Closing my eyes, I swallowed and saw Leah's profiled silhouette against the picturesque view of the sea. Three. Four. She was beautiful. I remembered her sweetness to me and her kindness. There was no gunshot when I took the rest of the pills. I went to sleep while watching my classmate peacefully standing in front of me above the shore.

Hours later, I woke up. I could not do it. I could not die. Like the alcohol, it was not enough. There was not enough liquor to take away the pain. There were not enough pills to take me out. *Why wouldn't He let me go?!*

Independence

I walked out of the post office and got into the car with a stack of envelopes in my hand. I shuffled through to the oversized, white one. I had a feeling about what it might be, but I was not sure until I saw the large, green letters on it: "UNC Charlotte ACCEPTANCE MATERIALS ENCLOSED"

I felt my eyes light up as I smiled so big, my face hardly contained it. "Oh, my God!" I said softly, "I got accepted."

Another smile faced me from the passenger seat. My mother saw me lifting the envelope for a closer look. Her smile made me happy. If she was feeling proud, maybe she was starting to remember.

I read through a ton of brochures and information packets towards the end of last summer. Some schools came off my wish list after discovering they did not offer my desired major. I gave up on the idea of going to California when I realized the severity of my mother's condition. Closer schools in border states showed interest in me over the years, but I did not want to go where I had not visited first. The only school left was UNC Charlotte.

I applied in October, five months earlier. I was confident in the high probability of being accepted. Still, receiving the envelope was a bit unexpected. If they checked my grades from the most recent semester, I doubt I would have gotten in. The acceptance packet and my mother's smile gave me hope. College was something to look forward to. It was also motivation for me to ensure my mother's healing. Her occupational therapy was going very well, thanks to a new therapist. Linda was a kind, red-headed woman. I told her about being accepted. She decided to partner with me in new goals for my mother. The number one priority was getting her ready to live independently before I left for college. Doctors removed her feeding tube before the holidays. My mother became more active in the kitchen. Sandra remembered recipes she learned as a child and could cook her preference of basic meals. A couple months passed before I completely trusted her in the kitchen by herself.

Another important step in the independence project was getting her back to old activities. Linda started by taking my mother to her old ceramics studio. I gave her the address and they went to a session while I was in school. The studio owner was very happy to see my mother. Surprisingly, pieces were still there from Mama's last visit almost a year ago. My mother did not remember them. The two stayed for a bit and she showed minor interest. Linda said ceramics could be something she tries at a later time. Typical errands were also part of the healing process. The trip to the post office was one. I also took her on grocery store runs. My mother's short-term memory was still a little sketchy. This was a great chance for her to practice making lists. She had to learn how to assess what she had and decide what she needed. All the exercises from her speech therapy helped with these cognitive skills. Sandra also had to get accustomed to using money again. There were times when she over or underestimated once she got to the store but there were ways around her mistakes.

Going to the store was a good introduction to my mother getting out of the house. We wanted Sandra to start going back to church, but it was a hurdle in her independence and presented several challenges. My mother did not remember Abundant Life. She thought she was still a member of the church she left after Grandmama died. Linda and I took a lot of time explaining her lost memories of being a Sunday school teacher and usher board member. Her face looked like she had a few flashbacks of what we were explaining. It helped me to remain hopeful. She quickly opened up to going. The next challenge was the possibility of overstimulation which caused most of her episodes. Our church was full of loud music and large crowds. Being surrounded by this for a long time could set her off. We decided to take her to similar environments to see how she responded. I took her to a family friend's son's baseball game. The Little League game was about two hours long with a decent-sized audience. Sandra sat quietly in the stands. She did not flinch at the crack of the bat or the roar of the crowd. When the game was over, the friend asked my mother if she had a good time. She responded positively.

"It was just nice to finally get out and go somewhere," she said. That's what I needed to hear. I told Linda about the game, and she felt confident my mother could handle the church service. We picked a Sunday. To be on the safe side, Linda would go with us to Sunday school and monitor my mother's reactions to determine whether we should stay for the remainder of the service.

That Sunday morning, my mother came out of her room wearing one of my favorite suits Mama used to wear to church. She looked like a woman who stepped out of the fitting room in a beautiful new outfit that just wasn't her style. It did not fit her body the way it once hugged Mama before the accident. She had on simple, black flats. Mama would have been in three-inch heels. Sandra's hair was now in a low afro clearly defining the shape of her skull. She seemed a little uncomfortable. Or maybe I was the uncomfortable one. Linda met us at Granddaddy's house.

"Oh, you look beautiful," Linda said to my mother.
This made her smile. I was really happy she was going with us. She always softened our space with the presence of her genuine heart. We took separate cars because if we stayed, Linda planned to leave after Sunday school.

One of my concerns was the people who would approach my mother when they saw her return. I knew they would be happy to see her back, but all the excitement directed at her might be too much. I discussed it with Linda before we came but it still weighed on my mind as we pulled into the parking lot. As soon as we got out of the car, I saw people looking. Linda immediately came over like a guard dog at a gate.

"Are you ready?" she asked both of us

"Oh, yeah," my mother replied. And with that, we walked towards the church doors.

The first person who noticed my mother was one of her fellow usher board members. Leon gently approached us with a smile. I was glad he was the first. Linda and I were able to explain our concerns to him. Leon said he would do his best to prevent my mother from being swarmed by a lot of people. He escorted us downstairs. Sunday school attendance was usually minimal, and this Sunday was no different. I went to the class for my age group. Linda stayed with my mother in the adult class. I had not gone to Sunday school in a while. It was nice to see my church friends. I wondered if everything was going okay but was not too worried knowing Linda was with her. We gathered when Sunday school was over. Linda enjoyed herself and was very pleased with how my mother handled everything and encouraged us to stay. We exchanged hugs and she went on her way.

A few people approached my mother before we went up to the sanctuary. The usher quickly seated us to avoid further well-intentioned greetings. The large church began to fill with people. I watched my mother closely. She seemed happy, swaying with the music and lifting her hands during worship. She even smiled a few times. Then our pastor approached the pulpit. He highlighted a few announcements before noticing my mother sitting in the congregation.

"Oh, my Lord," Pastor Moore said.

I knew it was coming. There was no way he would let the service pass without acknowledging her return.

"Stand up, Sister Sandra."

She grasped the pew in front of her with both hands and stood to her feet. The sanctuary erupted. People were clapping and shouting. The musicians played chords of solemn celebration. My mother lifted one hand high as she closed her eyes and shook her head. The moment was so touching, I wiped away tears. Finally, the congregation calmed themselves.

"That woman is a walking miracle," my pastor exclaimed.

Amens repeated across the sanctuary. He talked about her accident. I got a little annoyed when he incorrectly said she was hit by a semi-truck. I decided to correct him later. He said a lot of people were praying for her. Later Pastor Moore invited us to his family home for dinner.

Sandra made it through the long day. There were no episodes. The noise and the crowds did not bother her in the slightest. It seems she had a few flashes of memories about the church. She said some of the faces were familiar. The usher board members were most vivid in her mind which made sense. Mama spent a lot of time with them, and they were like a family. I was happy those images were still there and brought a little comfort. The comfort would be needed for the next hurdle.

The real test for my mother was spending the night at the house for the first time. Linda and I discussed it regularly. We knew it was going to be a major challenge. She had not been there since getting out of the hospital. Sandra never asked to go see it. Her response to the idea of going home was usually blank stares. As far as she was concerned, the house where she currently slept was her home. Linda told me not to be discouraged. Taking it slow would be key. We started with taking her to the house for a very short visit. I prepped the house before and made sure it was clean. I opened the curtains, so light came through the front. All the pictures and photo albums were visible. I hoped when she walked through the doors, maybe a piece of my Mama would come back. It was a nice idea but useless. My mother walked through the door and said nothing. We stayed for the duration of her session, walking through the house.

"How do you feel?" Linda asked. "Does anything look familiar?"

"I mean," Sandra began. "It's my house, I guess."

After about an hour, we returned to Granddaddy's house. We spent most of her weekly occupational therapy at the house on Gaynor. It was an opportunity for Sandra to exercise life skills in the place where she would ultimately live. She practiced cooking and doing laundry there. She watched a little television in the den. Several weeks passed before I heard her refer to the house as "my house." Hearing the words was encouraging.

Finally, the day came for her to spend a night there. I was so excited. The idea of my mother waking up in her room and in her own bed gave me hope. I felt it springing up inside me again. Maybe this was all she needed to get back to herself. I had this fantasy of my mother going to sleep and my Mama waking up, coming out of her bedroom, asking how long she was asleep, and what she missed in the past year. I eagerly packed my mother's bag for the night, placing a few extra clothing items in with the intention of some of it remaining at the house. The clothes would wait for her permanent return during this transition. She put up a little fuss about over-packing constantly reminding me this was just one night. Her reminders should have been my first clue.

We settled in the house for the night. All evening, she moved tentatively like a child inspecting her surroundings on her first sleepover. We ate dinner. I watched television with her in the den, hoping she would feel more comfortable. She took her medication while I watched. Then we went to our bedrooms. I wanted to close my small accordion door out of habit, but I knew it should remain open, at least until she fell asleep.

I sat on my bed and turned the TV down low. Her room was still dark, but I heard her fidgeting. Then, Sandra emerged in the doorway. She looked across the hall at me before going to the bathroom. Relief came over me. I heard her go further down the hallway. *What was she doing?* I decided to check the kitchen after seeing her return to her room. More relief came when I saw everything was as it should be. I went back to my room and sat on the bed.

I felt okay until she emerged in the doorway again. This time, she came to my door.

"We need to go home," she said, firmly.

"What?"

"We need to go home," she repeated.

"We are home," I said, just as firmly.

Her face was turning. I could not tell if she was scared, angry, or both. Either way, I did not want her to have an episode. I had to do something fast.

"What's wrong?" I asked.

"Ain't nothing wrong. We need to go home."

"Why?"

"Daddy home by himself," she replied.

"He's fine."

"How you know?!" she snapped

I knew I had to calm her down. She was not going to make it through the night if she did not feel safe. He was the only one that could keep this from escalating.

"Call him," I said.

I hated that I needed Granddaddy's help with her but I was not leaving. I was determined to sleep in my bed. She called him but I could not hear the conversation. Minutes later, she just hung up the phone and returned to bed without saying a word to me. I closed my door.

The next morning, we ate breakfast. She asked when we were going home while we sat at the table. I told her I would take her home when we were done. She quickly finished and got her bag. I put her in the car and drove down the street to Granddaddy's house at the stoplight. She walked in the door, content. I walked in the door, disgusted.

Prom & Graduation

As the end of my senior year quickly approached, I found myself taking care of Granddaddy and Mama full time. Granddaddy's cancer came back with a vengeance. We made several trips to the hospital. Every day, he woke up in excruciating pain. He was losing a lot of weight and a lot of strength. Granddaddy used to go out all the time. He went to church and visited friends but lately, he rarely got out of bed. At the beginning of the school year, I did not have to do much for him. I was able to focus on the tasks for my mother's healing. Now it was May and Granddaddy needed me just as much as she did.

Not going to prom was a real possibility. If Granddaddy needed around-the-clock care, there was no way I could go. My mother could not be alone with another sick person. I did not see any options until Aunt Barbara insisted, I should not miss such an important event in my high school years. She agreed to check in on them throughout the weekend. Then my favorite cousin, Chanel, offered to be my date. Going to prom with my cousin was not what I imagined but I was touched by the sentiment. I agreed and made the plans.

The prom was on a Friday night. I headed straight to the salon when I got out of school at 12:30 that afternoon. For an hour and a half, I sat waiting for the hairdresser before she even started the four-hour process on my hair. Anger torched my face with every passing minute. When she was done, the hairstyle was less than impressive but there was no time to complain. I rushed out to my sister who offered to rent a car for me. My heart sank when I arrived at her house and there was no car. With no credit card to secure the rental, she offered her car instead. The catch was I could not use the car until later that night. I did not want to drive Granddaddy's old

LeBaron tonight. Mama's Buick still sat in his yard but it was not drivable. There was no other transportation. I went back to Granddaddy's house and sat in the den in tears.

I prepared myself, once again, for the possibility of not going to my senior prom. The tears were still falling when I heard a sweet, familiar voice.

"Quala. What's wrong?"

My cousin, Vanessa, stood in the den doorway. I looked up to Aunt Dorothy's youngest daughter since I was a little girl. She was everything I wanted to be when I grew up. Vanessa was a beautiful, smart and sophisticated young woman. Seven years earlier, she made me feel like a princess as a flower girl in her wedding. I wanted to walk down the aisle with the same class my cousin emitted with her presence. Vanessa was an Air Force Officer which limited the times I saw her. I figured she was home on leave because seeing her tonight was very unexpected, but very much needed. There was no point in hiding my sadness.

"It's my prom night," I said through tears. I explained how my plans were falling through all day. Vanessa listened.

Then, in her authoritative, Air Force officer tone, she said, "No, you're going to your prom." Her family check-in visit was a mission of epic proportion.

First, she attempted to rent a car for me but nothing was available. She decided to take me herself. Unfortunately, with the time wasted at the salon and the rental car fiasco, I could not get to Chanel. I was okay with going by myself. After checking on Granddaddy and making dinner, I gave my mother her medicine. The night was flying by. I threw on my dress from the Miss WPAL pageant and tried to salvage some sort of hairstyle. Vanessa took a picture of me by the refrigerator before driving me to prom. People were leaving as we arrived. She dropped me off and told me she would return in about forty-five minutes, right before prom ended.

There was still a crowd at the Officer's Club. I tried to get the traditional prom picture, but the line was so long and I did not want to spend the little time I had waiting. A few friends said hello but there was only one friend I was looking for. Veronica was the most talkative person I knew and the most fun. We had been attached by the hip since before Thanksgiving break. She was aware of my struggles at home but always made me focus on enjoying the time I was not there. We bought a ticket to every movie premiering that year and went to all of the senior events together including cut day at the beach. I went to her house party. She came to my rowdy spades game. We spent so much time together, spending prom weekend with her just seemed fitting. Our plan was a short weekend trip to a penthouse I saved all year for. We would hang out with some guy friends, and I would focus on just enjoying being a teenager.

I found Veronica just before Vanessa returned. My cousin took both of us to her big, beautiful house where we changed. Then she drove us back to my sister's place to pick up her car. I said my thank you's and goodbyes and we pulled off. We headed to Mama's house to pick up my packed bag for the weekend. On the way, I vented to my friend about how my prom had fallen apart.

"Well, that's over now," Veronica interrupted. "You're still going away for the weekend. So, we're gonna forget about all that and we're going to have some fun."

She was right. I shifted my focus to what was ahead and tried to put the events of the day out of my mind but they still nagged at me. Mama's accident robbed me of another milestone. I wanted someone to help me get it back. I needed a hero. Turning a corner, I realized exactly who I wanted my hero to be.

"You know what," I said. "I have to make a phone call."
There was no time to wait until we got to the house. I pulled into the next gas station and went to the phone booth. The receiver nearly slipped through my hands as I picked it up, put in the quarter, and

dialed his number. Only a few rings passed before I heard his strong, soothing voice.

"Hello."

David and I saw each other only once since the beginning of the school year when Veronica invited him to the spades game at my house. We avoided even the slightest physical contact but could not take our eyes off each other. Just being in the same room together awakened every feeling we pushed down deep for over a year. He worked during the day and went to school at night. He also had a new girlfriend. I wanted to respect his relationship the way he respected my decision not to have sex. I purposely distanced myself from him the entire first semester of school. But, I missed my friend.

I reached out to David on the Monday before prom. I told him about my plans for the weekend and invited him to join us. There were no expectations or hidden agendas. It would just be a group of friends having fun and making memories. He wanted to say yes but he just reunited with his girlfriend and also had to work on Saturday afternoon. He said he would still think about it. He was on the fence when he called me before getting my hair done. I was going to let it go but after all the disappointments of the day, I needed something to go my way.

"Hey," I said. "I thought I would give you one last chance before we leave."

I almost felt bad for taking advantage of David. I knew it was near impossible for him to say no to me, especially if he sensed I needed him. A few moments of silence passed before he responded.

"Man, bump it. I'm going. Give me twenty minutes."

"Okay." I hung up the phone and got back in the car.

We headed to my house to get my weekend bag. I was excited as we walked through the back door. Veronica sat in the den while I quickly packed my things in my bedroom. We laughed about how surprised the other two guys would be when they saw David in the car. I heard Veronica talking as I opened my dresser drawer. Slowly, her voice began to muffle, and the silence grew thick. I walked into the den. She was still talking. I tried to cover the fact that her voice was muted. The silence was familiar. It was the same as the night I prepared for the Miss North Charleston High pageant. Here I was, again, getting ready for another milestone and Mama was not here. I walked back to my bedroom before the silence overwhelmed me. Quickly throwing the last of the clothes in the bag, I told Veronica I was ready.

The excitement reignited once I pulled into David's driveway. He was waiting for me at the door. As he approached the car with his overnight bag, his smile made me exhale.

"Wassup?" he smoothly asked.

I let go of all the frustration from the day. My hero was here. We went to meet Veronica's friends and got on the road. A two-hour drive to Columbia, SC was ahead of us. It was dark on Interstate 26. The hour was late. Veronica fell asleep in the passenger seat. I fixed my eyes on the head-lit road in front of me, completely alert. My mind settled on the one laying in the back seat. I thought he was asleep until about an hour into the drive.

"Hey. Are you alright?" David asked.

"Yeah, I'm good." Had I drifted off? I didn't think so.

"You sure?" He pressed.

"Yes, I'm fine."

"OK." I felt his hand on my arm. He was awake during the entire drive.

We arrived at the penthouse a little before 2 a.m. We were all ecstatic. We walked through, inspecting our accommodations.

"This is nice," Veronica's friend said.

It was true. The penthouse was a teenager's dream. I was finally happy. Then, I went to the bathroom. Horror gripped me as I looked down in disbelief. It was prom night, I was at a penthouse for the weekend, and my freaking period was on. With no pads packed, I was completely unprepared. Thankfully, everyone agreed we should go to an all-night grocery store to stock the kitchen. My goal was to discreetly get what I needed while we were there. That plan failed. The paper bag I had stood out like a red ball in a cotton field. Veronica's friend went straight for it.

"What you got in a paper bag? Some pads or something?"

I shot him a look so fierce, it wiped the smile off his face. "Yes!" I snapped, "I bought some big, extra-long, overnight pads and I ain't shame." I stomped to the car.

"Damn right!" Veronica said in solidarity.

We jumped in the front seat and closed our doors. The three guys stood outside, looking at each other. After a few seconds, one of them tentatively opened a back door. They quietly sat in the back seat.

"So, who's cooking breakfast in the morning?" I asked.

The awkwardness was broken, and we laughed all the way back to the penthouse.

Sleeping arrangements were simple and tasteful. Veronica's friends were upstairs. She and I were downstairs. David jokingly joined us. We all settled in for the night. I laid in the darkness with my eyes wide open. I remembered I had not said my nightly prayers. The words I wrote years ago repeated like a chorus in my head. Usually, if I forgot to say them or the hour was late, I would recite the prayer in bed. Tonight, I could not say the words.

I looked at David lying beside me, wishing Veronica was not on the other side. I thought about getting up and going into the living room. Maybe David would realize I was not there, and he would get up to find me. He would sit next to me, ask me what's wrong, and would gently take my hand as he had done so many times before. I would tell him how tired I was, how scared I was. I would tell him how much I had lost. Then, he would remind me of the girl he knew. He'd remind me of my strength and talent and hold me through my quiet tears. I desperately wanted him to hold me but didn't move. I turned my head to look at the forms in the darkness. Then, I felt David's hand again.

"Go to sleep," he whispered.

I nestled close to him and finally, closed my eyes.

***

Graduation was in two weeks. I struggled with the idea of inviting Daddy. After Mama's accident, I felt it was my responsibility to make him suffer the way she did. Inviting him felt like a betrayal to her. Still, something in me wanted him there. I felt like he did not deserve the invitation, but he was still my father. The inner turmoil angered me. It wasn't fair to have to make this decision with everything else going on in my life. I decided on an unleashing compromise. I called his house and left a message.

"Hey. This is Quala. Your daughter," speaking as snarky as possible. "So, I guess you should know that I'm graduating on June 3rd at three o'clock. Not that you deserve to come since you haven't been here for anything else. But at least now, you can't say you didn't know. So come if you want. I don't care. Okay. Bye."

I felt grown and powerful saying what I said. I was everything I thought Mama would have taken pleasure in concerning my father. After hanging up, I felt like an idiot. Later, my sister Tasha told me she heard the message. She said Daddy was very hurt. Her disappointment cut me, but I was so emotionally numb from the past year's pain, I barely felt it.

North Charleston High provided an official count after prom. The 1995 school year began with 303 seniors and ended with 293 graduates. I wondered how close I was to being in the group of ten who didn't make it. Mrs. Pavlisko was responsible for this. Failing English was certain. All of the missed assignments went through my mind as I approached the gym for the ceremony rehearsal. An administrator stood at the entrance. Every senior stopped to see if their name was on the administrator's list. If your name was not on the list, there was no point for you to enter and you were turned away. Seconds felt like hours while I waited for them to find my name. I was almost embarrassed knowing how shocked my friends would be.

"There you are," the lady said. "We know you're here."

I smiled and walked into the gym. My only thought was about Mrs. Pavlisko. My diploma was a debt I owed to her understanding.

Graduation was two days later and a hectic day for me. Burke High School's ceremony was downtown at 10:00 a.m. K'Lani and I had talked about going to each other's graduation since we were in middle school. We were concerned our ceremonies might fall on the same day. Thankfully, they fell at different times which allowed us to plan our days. I was so excited to see my best friend walk across the stage. After the last name was called, I rushed out of the auditorium. I was happy to run into K'Lani's sister so she would know I was there. We chatted briefly about my ceremony before I got in the car and drove home.

It was a few minutes past noon. Less than two hours remained before graduates were expected at the North Charleston Coliseum. I went back to Granddaddy's house first. My mother was there alone because he was in the hospital for a week. She was sitting in the living room when I walked in. I had a weird flashback of Granddaddy sitting in the same armchair on the day Cole was sentenced. I shook the picture from my mind and checked in. I reminded my mother that Aunt Barbara would come by to bring her to the ceremony. I was leaving to get ready at the house.

"You going to see Daddy?" she asked.

"Huh?" I was thrown by the question.

"When are you going to see Daddy?" She was angry. My hesitation triggered her.

I had been to the hospital almost every day since he was admitted, including the day before.

"I don't see how there will be time. Graduation is at three o'clock and visiting hours end early today."

She stood up. "Well, go before."

"I can't. I have to be at the coliseum at two."

"Well, I'm going to see Daddy."

"When?" I asked, "What about graduation?"

"Don't nobody give a damn about no graduation!"

I stood there, looking at her. I looked into her eyes. She was telling the truth. My mother's only concern, on my graduation day, was her Daddy. I knew Aunt Barbara would make sure she came but her heart would not be there. I wanted to say something to make her remember. I wanted this day to be as important to her as it was to me, but it was pointless. All I could do was walk out.

My mother's words repeated in my head as I changed into my white suit. Shaking my head, I replaced them with images of my friends cheering for me when my name was called. Getting ready in Mama's house, in my bedroom, was supposed to help the day feel like it should feel. I tried to imagine how the day would have gone if she was here. I looked towards Mama's bedroom door and almost saw her smile. She would have rushed me from K'Lani's graduation, back to the house, and then out the door, so she could drop me off at the ceremony. I picked up my freshly ironed, gold cap and gown off the bed. This was not the graduation day I imagined.

The entrance for graduates led to tunnels below the coliseum. Mrs. Pavlisko's generosity popped into my head. I wanted to thank her, but the organized chaos left no room for disruption. Ceremony volunteers quickly led me to my place in line. I chatted with Elliott, standing behind me with whom I shared many honors classes over the years. We laughed about our high school journeys. Then we saw Mrs. Lavely passing out the Teacher Cadet cords. My insides began to cringe knowing Elliott was in the class with me. He said what I knew was coming.

"Oh, you need to get your cord."

I knew I was not going to get one, but I panicked. I smiled and walked over to Mrs. Lavely. The sad look on her face already said the words she so sweetly whispered in my ear.

"You had to pass the class to wear one."

I nodded my head and smiled. "I know."

She hugged me before I walked back to my place in line. I was so embarrassed. I knew I would have to answer the inevitable question.

"What happened? Where's your cord?"

"You had to pass the class to get one," I repeated.

"Oh."

I saw the shock on his face. I was the only person from the class without the distinctive decoration. My heart sank as I realized there was nothing on my gown to show for those years of hard work and honors classes. There were no stoles. No cords. My naked neck was proof of how I allowed the accident to put a line through everything I accomplished.

"Well, you're getting your diploma," Elliott said. "That's what matters."

"Right." I forced a smile as we moved into our places.

Graduation went fast. The new mayor of North Charleston gave the keynote address, but our class president's speech brought us to our feet. Afterward, no one would remember what either one said. We sat anxiously waiting for the presentation of our diplomas. When it was time, we stood row by row like we rehearsed. I heard my name yelled from the stands when my row got in line.

Finally, I walked on stage. My full name was called. I flashed a big smile and put two fingers in the peace sign. I saw one of my friends and fellow graduates laughing in the first row. Then, I turned to receive my diploma. My heart was full when I saw the woman placing the cover in my hand. The first principal of Buist Academy, who was now a school superintendent. Miss Murray remembered me and gave me a huge hug. I felt like school had come full circle.

The blue faux-leather diploma holders we received on stage were empty. Immediately following the ceremony, we were directed back to the tunnels where our diplomas were placed inside. This signaled the end of our time at North Charleston High School. I could hear our class song, *U Will Know*, in my head. Our diplomas were grouped alphabetically at tables. I found mine and was elated when I saw it. Somehow, I still managed to receive the gold emblem indicating the college preparatory curriculum I had taken my entire high school career. I thought I would receive a regular diploma after I dropped the required pre-calculus class to save me from suspension during the attendance fiasco. A little piece of something I was sure I lost, was returned. They placed my gold sealed diploma in the holder, and I headed for the door.

A mass of families waited for the graduates at the exit. I had been looking forward to this since going to Chanel's graduation, the year before. The idea of all these people waiting reminded me of fans waiting to see their favorite celebrity. It was the one moment I was waiting for, but it did not last long. Two of my sisters quickly whisked me away. Tasha and Shawn were waiting for me at the exit doors. They pulled me away so fast, I did not get a chance to see anyone or say thank you to others for coming.

We went straight to Granddaddy's house. My mother was there with some of my aunts, my cousin Vanessa, and other family members. I hoped to see Willie but I was happy his sister, Thelma, was there. Everyone seemed happy for me but no one was happier than my sisters. I was drawn to their excitement. They celebrated the milestone with balloons and picture taking. Then they were ready to take me to dinner. Everything happened so fast. I allowed the whirlwind of my sister's celebration to make me ignore how the rest of my family, who came to support me, was being left out. Auntie Thelma and Vanessa made this very clear when they pulled me to the side.

"So, where y'all going to eat?" Auntie Thelma asked.

"I'm not sure," I said. "I don't think they decided."

I began to feel anxious. My sisters were ready to go. Their mother and grandmother had elected to stay in the car. They were waiting outside.

"What about yo' Mama?"

I cringed when anyone called her that. "Oh, of course, she can come." It sounded bizarre when I said it.

"She's your mother, Quala," Vanessa interjected. "There shouldn't be a question."

Auntie Thelma cosigned. "That's right. We all came to support you too."

They were right. I should have said something, but I was not strong enough.

The rest of my family was gracious when I left with my sisters. I felt horrible. Their grandmother chose the Old Country Buffet restaurant. I hated that place, but I figured I deserved it for the way I handled the situation. I was glad when dinner was over.

Later that evening, I met up with Shelly and Trena. The three of us had been inseparable since the New Year. We got something to eat and hung out for the rest of the night. They made me laugh and reminded me how I was supposed to be feeling as a seventeen-year-old. Once again, my friends saved the day. High school was officially over. This was where real life was supposed to begin, but not for me. Real-life had started more than a year ago, and death was just around the corner.

The Sequel

"Your grandfather wants to see you," Tanya said.

It was a couple of nights before graduation. I waited outside his hospital room, walking the floor, thinking of the last time I was there. A year ago, my mother was in a different wing. Everything in the hospital seemed different until my distant cousin came to get me. I followed her to his room. It was dark. Tubes were coming from his arm and nose. The machine monitoring his pulse lit up the left side of his face. I watched him from the door. This was too familiar. I stepped closer. There were a few people in the room and one of them told him I was there. He tilted his head and looked at me. I almost saw pride in his eyes. I hoped I did. Granddaddy never said he was proud of me over the past year. He turned his head back. One tear fell from his eye as he whispered.

"What's gonna happen to that boy?" He asked, staring at the ceiling.

Cole had been at Lieber Correctional for over a year. Granddaddy never gave up on getting his sentence reduced. He diligently worked with an attorney since the hearing. I saw the paperwork and heard a few conversations. The more time passed, it became increasingly clear nothing would change any time soon. Hearing Granddaddy ask the question made me realize he would never see Cole outside of prison walls again. Looking at Granddaddy's tears in the hospital bed, I prayed Cole said he was sorry at some point over the past year. If not, it was too late. On my way out of the hospital room, I heard my grandfather saying, "I wanna go home. I wanna go home."

Granddaddy got his wish. The Sunday after graduation, I went to church alone. My mother only went back a few times since her first service. Lately, she wanted to spend most of her time at home

149

with Granddaddy. Aunt Barbara took her to pick him up from the hospital. The house was filled with people when I returned in the afternoon. Granddaddy laid in his room but it was different. His big four-post bed was replaced with a hospital bed. The nurse stood by the nightstand, explaining something to the other women in the room, including Aunt Barbara. No one noticed me walk past the door and through the kitchen to Cole's room. I wanted to remain unseen, but I knew they should be aware of my presence. The nurse met me in the living room. She introduced herself and we sat down at the dining room table.

"Your aunt said you would be the one here most of the time," Nurse Janie said.

"Yes," I answered.

"Well, they can explain most of this to you. But there are a few things you need to know."

The nurse pulled out a folder with the word "Hospice" on the cover. The term sounded familiar from commercials. All I associated with Hospice was the end of life. She began to talk about feeding schedules and breath monitoring. Different nurses were scheduled throughout the week. A stack of paperwork with procedures and phone numbers lined the table. Janie stressed not calling 911 if Granddaddy stopped breathing. My first call should be to Hospice. Aunts Barbara, Debbie, and Mina came out of the room. They talked with Nurse Janie a little before she left while I sat at the dining room table.

This was the same scene from a year ago with Mama. School was out. In a bedroom was the sickness requiring round-the-clock care. The nurse was leaving. Another freaking folder lay on the table. Aunt Barbara talked about when she could be here and what I should do. I did not want to do this again. My heart began to race. I lifted my elbows to the table and placed my forehead in my hands.

"You alright, Quala," someone asked.

I did not know who was talking to me. I didn't care. I told them what they wanted to hear. "Yeah, I'm fine," I said as I lifted my head. "I'm just gonna go back to Cole's room for a minute."

I quickly got up and went back to the room. My body was numb, and my mind went blank. I had to calm myself down.

"I'm seventeen," I whispered.

Tears fell from my face to the hardwood floor. Graduation was less than twenty-four hours ago. It seemed insignificant and long forgotten. I wanted to throw or break something. The walls were just about to close in until I looked out the window. The bush in the front garden was green and full. Past McCant's station, I could see the Mixon Avenue intersection where the stoplight indicated the end of Liberty Hill. I looked out the window and forced myself to breathe.

"You can do this. You can do this." I got up and walked back to the front of the house.

Granddaddy's daughters, Debbie, Barbara, and my mother stood in the living room. His oldest sister, Auntie Mina, went back to her house next door. Aunt Debbie was leaving but planned to return later for the night watch. Until then, Aunt Barbara would stay for a few hours. I grabbed the folder off the table to take it into Granddaddy's room. I opened the door and stepped down from the living room. His room was so dark. I placed the folder on his dresser across from where he slept. The room felt so weighted like cancer had taken a form and filled the walls. I turned and stepped out.

Aunt Barbara and my mother were sitting in the living room. The house was quiet. Aunt Barbara said it would not last long. Visitors were coming and keeping the house clean was my number one priority. This too was familiar. I remembered how Aunt Pine came last summer. I worked hard to maintain all the deep cleaning she did. I considered it a way to show my heart's gratitude. Keeping the house clean would not be a problem.

I went to the kitchen to assess the grocery situation. The cabinets were fully stocked with canned goods and a prepared meal warmed on the stove. I opened the fridge and saw some cans of 7Up soda and Ensure supplement drinks which would be Granddaddy's meals when he could not eat. I ended up buying more from CVS the next day, as Granddaddy didn't eat the dinner Auntie Mina prepared.

Early Monday morning, I checked on Granddaddy. My mother was already in the living room. A new nurse came later that morning. She stayed long enough to check Granddaddy's vitals and monitor his breathing pattern. He was breathing normally and fairly lucid. Though he could not sit up in bed, he was still able to drink from the straw I placed in the glass for him. I held it to his mouth while he drank only a little. My Grandfather didn't say a word to me.

There was one person who desperately needed to hear him say something. Mr. Brickman was Granddaddy's attorney for a long time. Their business relationship was cased in loyalty that superseded attorney-client privilege. Mr. Brickman was a confidant. He called the house daily when Granddaddy came home. I knew they were close, but it was clear these were business calls. On Monday, he was able to speak to Granddaddy for a little while. He would not be so lucky in the days following but it did not stop him from calling.

"It is very important that I speak with your grandfather," he insisted.

I heard the urgency in his voice. "I'm sorry," I said. "I mean, I could hold the phone up to his ear, but I don't think he'll respond."

For a second, I think Mr. Brickman actually considered the option. He seemed to need only the slightest indication of affirmation or refute. I wondered what was so important. Why did he need to speak with him so badly? Ultimately, he had to let it go and surrender to the inevitable.

Granddaddy was fading. By Tuesday, there was no use in trying to have a conversation with him. He was conscious but slept through most of the day. His brothers and sisters came to visit him, one by one. Granddaddy was very close to his siblings, especially his brothers, Jimmy and Willie. They shared a deep bond of friendship and duty to protect their family name. I was not surprised to see them quietly weeping at their brother's bedside.

A mainstay in Granddaddy's room was Aunt Debbie. She came for the overnight hours, just as she said she would. She sat in a chair at the side of the bed with the lamp on. Her arms rested on the bed, against the rails, cradling her head as she slept. It did not look very comfortable. I watched her one night. Dressed for her job, she would immediately go to work after leaving her father's bedside. Uncle Jerome, Aunt Debbie's husband, provided a wake-up call for her every morning. I answered the phone quickly. When I heard his voice, I gave her the phone. She simply said, "OK," and hung up. Then she gathered her things and quietly left.

Aunt Debbie reminded me of Aunt Pine. Both women helped where they could with no questions asked and no recognition required. They didn't cleverly seek validation by talking about how they had done so much for someone. They never spoke of what they did for others at all. Their service spoke kindness and forgiveness to whom it was rendered and to the world around them. Watching Aunt Debbie on those mornings as the sun rose, made me see love in a whole new way.

Uncle Jerome's wake-up calls sometimes woke Granddaddy up before Aunt Debbie. She jumped at the sound we heard constantly throughout the night.

"May! May!" Granddaddy was calling out for his cousin.

May was a distant cousin known for her elegant style and fancy taste. She and Mama were quite close despite the age difference. Cousin May was a little closer to Granddaddy's age but still younger. They were not around each other much. She lived nearby on Deas Hill. How we were related was still a mystery. I just counted her as another one of the endless cousins all black people seem to have.

Granddaddy began calling for May on Monday night. For four days, he yelled her name over and over. May was on his lips when he woke up and when he fell asleep. Finally, we contacted her, and she came. He was yelling her name when she walked through the door.

"Hey! Hey!" she yelled back. "I'm here. I hear you been calling for me. I'm right here."

I hoped he was as happy to see her, as I was. He yelled her name a few more times and then quieted down. I stepped away when she started talking to him. The words said in that room were private. A little while passed before she came out. Cousin May had the Smalls family's ability to give respectful courtesy with the slightest bit of underlying disdain. She and Aunt Barbara exchanged basic pleasantries like the distant cousins they were. After which, she proudly got in her Cadillac and drove away.

Granddaddy continued to call for May until late Friday afternoon. By Saturday morning, he stopped speaking altogether. It was time to accept the inevitable. I was not so sure if my mother started this process. Sandra did not fully grasp the severity of his condition. She was happy Granddaddy was home, going about her day, as usual, eating, watching television, and speaking with visitors. I stayed close when she went into Granddaddy's room, peeking in only if it seemed she was in there too long. She never cried. Whenever I peeped in, she was sitting by the bed or adjusting the covers. With each passing day, I deeply feared what this loss would do to her. I also feared the strong possibility I would be there when the inevitable happened.

All week long, I made myself scarce when Aunt Barbara or a nurse was there. Most of the time, I was with my friends, Shelly and Trena. I prepared myself for the news of his death each time I walked through the door. When there was no news, I prayed he would make it through the night. I wanted him to make it through the next twenty-four hours. Nurses were off duty for the weekend. Aunt Debbie and Aunt Barbara needed a break. I desperately tried to find coverage for Sunday morning, but no one was available.

When the last visitor left on Saturday evening, I was alone with my mother and Granddaddy. After dinner, I settled Sandra in her room. I turned the TV off in the living room and went to sit with Granddaddy. Sitting in the chair closest to the living room door, I watched him breathe. For the first time, the unassailable effects of cancer stared at me with no remorse. The man in the bed was a shell of the grandfather I knew. Granddaddy was a strong, built man with a face full of wisdom and vitality. The shriveled frame lying in front of me did not have the hands that opened the doors of Green Temple Missionary Baptist Church and set up instruments and stacked Bibles for Sunday school. It did not have the legs that walked the gardens, plucking vegetables for Grandmama's dinners. Cancer had eaten away the bones of a man I loved and respected.

As I sat there watching him breathe, his eyes were closed. His mouth was open. Seconds passed between each breath. A chill fell over the room. I rubbed my hands against my arms to warm them. Glancing back at the bed, I realized Granddaddy's feet were exposed. The blanket and sheet were pulled off to the side. I peeked out the door to see if my mother had come out of her room. No one was there. The air in the room shifted and was colder when I got up to walk towards the bed.

"Granddaddy," I said quietly, waiting for a response
Then, he exhaled. It was one, dull, and long breath. I slowly reached for the sheet and blanket. My hands grazed his feet as I covered them. They were as cold as ice. Looking back up to his face, I wanted to touch him but fear gripped me. So, I stepped back, listening for one more breath. Hearing it made me finally exhale.

The next morning, I went to his room, nervous about what I would find. He was still there. There were more seconds between each audible breath, but he was still breathing. I made a futile attempt to give him some fluids. I knew it was pointless, but I had to try. It was like putting a straw in a doll's mouth. The room was still cold on that warm June day. Backing away to the door, I looked directly at his eyes. Though they were closed, I said the words anyway.

"I love you, Granddaddy." I stepped into the living room and closed the door.

My mother sat on the sofa. I couldn't tell if she was oblivious or in denial. This would be his last day. I wanted to tell her to go and be with her Daddy, but my instinct said it was not a good idea. Charleston's heat and humidity were making her drowsy. She barely kept her eyes open.

"You know what," I said, "people are gonna be coming by when they get out of church. Let's go lay down while we have a chance."

"Yeah, you right." She stood up and looked in Granddaddy's room. I prayed he let out a breath for her.

"Daddy, I'm going to lie down."

She closed the door. Her face said nothing mournful or fearful as we walked down the hall. I waited to see her go into her room and settle on her bed. Then, I went into Cole's room, closed the door and put my head on the pillow. Sleep came easy but did not last long. My eyes opened at the knock on Cole's door and a woman's gentle voice calling my name.

"Quala? Quala?" I recognized Granddaddy's pastor.

"Yes ma'am," I answered.

"We need you to come here," she said calmly. "I can't find a pulse on your grandfather."

Saying Goodbye

I stepped down into Granddaddy's room and closed the door behind me. The face in the bed looked the same but somehow void. Careful not to get too close, I took a few steps forward. His room was different. The Charleston heat fought the stale breeze of the fans. I listened for a few seconds. Nothing. My mouth opened to call his name, but I knew there was no use. Granddaddy was gone. The air had carried him away.

On the dresser across from the bed lay the Hospice folder. I reached for it and put on the necessary brave face before opening the door. My mother was waiting. There was no need to speak. Reality sank in, causing her legs to buckle. She reached for the wall with one hand and her forehead with the other. Her mouth was open but no sound came out. She was like a baby holding in air before exhaling the soul-shaking cries. I caught her before she hit the floor. Granddaddy's pastor helped me lift her up and onto the sofa. My heart ached for her. This was a hard blow. My comfort was not wanted. She pushed me away like all babies do when the only person they want is their parent. The pastor sat on the sofa with her. I picked up the folder I dropped while lifting her and went to the dining room table.

The instructions were clear. Call Hospice first. I found the number and made the call. It wasn't long before the nurse arrived. She was a short, dark-skinned woman with glasses. I led her to the room through the kitchen door. My mother did not see the nurse come out of the room. I was afraid it might make things worse. A few minutes passed before she came back into the kitchen. The nurse began to take notes without saying a word. It was like I was not even there. I looked directly at her with razor eyes, hoping she would feel me waiting for her to interact with the comfort and empathy they talked about in the folder.

Tired of waiting, I finally spoke. "Uh, excuse me. Is he…?"

She looked up at me to respond, "Oh…yes, he's deceased." She looked down and returned to her paperwork.

Really? I thought to myself. This woman pissed me off. *Did I look too young to understand or was I just insignificant to her job?* I could not spend too much time in this anger. There was too much to be done and people who needed to be told, immediately. I left the nurse at the table with her important paperwork. Then, I picked up the phone and called Aunt Barbara, but Uncle Julius said she was not home from church yet. The next place to look for her was only a block up the street, but I decided to go get Auntie Mina first. I asked the pastor to stay with my mother while I went next door. She kindly agreed.

Delivering this information to people so close to my grandfather felt weird. Knowing I was the last one in the room was a bit daunting. I dreaded this responsibility all week long. My friend, Shelly, knew how bad I did not want to be there when he died. She warned me this would happen, but I just hoped to be spared. As I walked into Auntie Mina's yard, the gravity of what I had to do hit me.

Her big door was open. I saw her moving around through the screen door. She was still in her church clothes. I knocked on the door.

"Auntie Mina?"

She stopped in her living room and looked at me. "Oh, hey Quala. Come on in," she said smiling as she opened the door.

Nervously, I walked in. I tried to smile back but couldn't. This was his oldest sister. She'd buried siblings before, and she was about to bury another. Maybe that's why she recognized the look on my face.

"Did he pass?" she asked.

"Yes ma'am."

"OK," she said with a forced but understanding smile. "Let me just get my keys."

She moved as if she was doing routine housework. Auntie Mina was always focused. She handled life as if she was prepared for everything, including death. We stepped outside and she locked the front door. I walked her over.

She and Granddaddy's pastor exchanged greetings. I thanked her for staying with my mother and told her we would be calling soon with arrangement details. After the pastor left, Auntie Mina stayed with my mother while I went to get Aunt Barbara. Being held in Auntie Mina's arms was more comforting for my mother. They were on the sofa when I left. Each time I walked by the kitchen door, I thought about my grandfather's body still lying in the hospital bed. I walked by quickly.

Aunt Barbara was going to be a little more difficult to tell. I wondered if she would blame me for being asleep when he died. I felt the same fear when I had to tell Granddaddy about Little. I saw Aunt Barbara's car in her cousin's yard, a house I had never been to before. Her cousin, Cookie, answered when I knocked on the door.. She said hello but knew who I was there for. Aunt Barbara was in clear view from where I stood. She was relaxed in this place. Unlike Auntie Mina, Aunt Barbara had changed out of her church clothes. She immediately knew something was wrong when she looked at me.

"Is he gone?"

I was scared when I got there and horribly uncomfortable. Panicked, not knowing what to say, I simply repeated what the pastor said to me.

"I can't get a pulse." She stood up and gathered her purse and other items.

"You ready for this, Barb," Cookie reassured her.

"That's right. I knew it was coming," Aunt Barbara replied.

"I'm praying," Cookie said.

They said goodbyes and we walked to the car. I got into the passenger seat but wondered if I should drive when I looked over at my aunt. She was shaking. Her breathing seemed more like hyperventilating.

"I can do this. I can do this. Oh, God. I can do this," she repeated to herself.

"You okay?" I asked. "Do you want me to drive?"

"No, I can make it a block across the street."

She did. When we arrived, the Hospice nurse was still there. She relayed minor information to Auntie Mina. Aunt Barbara went ahead to the living room. I had to walk past that kitchen door again. Aunt Barbara did not know what was on the other side but I did.

All three women were in there when I finally walked through the kitchen into the dining room. The door was cracked open. I saw them surrounding the bed. Then, they began to wail. It was loud and deep. Their cries were unexpected. Aunt Barbara and Auntie Mina were two of the hardest women I knew. They were matriarchs who took care of their families while taking the beatings life handed them. What I heard coming out of that room was pain. It was like the stories I read about ancient female mourning rituals where the women spent hours or even days crying and wailing over the dead bodies of loved ones. My mother and my aunts did not stay in the room for long. They came out wiping their tears, standing tall, and ready to get down to business. I sat at the dining room table where they joined me. The pain that unified them was quickly put to the side as the silent but clear question arose. Who is going to be in charge?

The power struggle began with the very first decision to be made. I told them that according to Hospice, we needed to call the funeral home to get Granddaddy's body. North Area Funeral Home was part of the fabric of Liberty Hill. The family owners knew everyone in the community. One of Granddaddy's old friends was the founder. They buried Grandmama. I quietly agreed with Auntie Mina that they were the obvious choice. Aunt Barbara had something else in mind.

"I think he should go to Suburban," she said.

Suburban was another black-owned funeral home in a different predominantly black neighborhood. Auntie Mina was appalled.

"The Hiltons have known Sammie for years. It wouldn't be right to send him somewhere else."

"I just don't want them people in our business," Aunt Barbara retorted.

"What business? I don't..." Auntie Mina stopped. "You know what? Go 'head. Whatever you want."

Aunt Barbara looked at me and firmly said, "Suburban." Something about this was too easy, but I didn't ask any questions. I went to the Hospice nurse and told her to make the call.

There were three more people who needed to be told immediately. Aunt Barbara agreed to call her two sisters. I wanted to be the one to tell Cole. He called a few times in the past week. The last time we spoke, I explained how Granddaddy could not talk and was barely conscious. I heard the fear in my brother's voice as reality set in. The man he knew as Daddy, was dead. I was ready to make the call until Aunt Barbara stopped me. Prisons had a process which did not allow minors to relay information to prisoners. I was only seventeen. Cole could not hear it from me.

The funeral home was on its way to pick up the body. I did not want to be there. The idea of seeing strangers place Granddaddy into a bag and then shoving it into the back of a vehicle was too much. The image was not one I wanted etched in my memory. I asked Aunt Barbara if they could handle everything else. More people needed to be notified but they would make those calls. Funeral arrangements could be made in the morning. She encouraged me to go and I gladly took the offer. The hearse pulled up just as I walked out the door.

I ran to the phone booth on the corner and called Shelly. My heart calmed down when I heard my friend's voice. I wasted no time.

161

"Well, you were right," I said. "I was there."

"He died today?" She asked.

"Yep. Girl, the hearse just came to take his body. I cannot be here. Please ask your momma if I can come over."

Her mother was happy to have me. I needed to be around Shelly and Trena. Hiding my feelings or being strong was not necessary around them. I could be my complete self. The truth was my complete self was very afraid of the coming days.

After a few hours at Shelly's house, I returned to my grandfather's late Sunday evening. One of my worst fears was sleeping in a house where I witnessed death come in and take someone. Sleeping was not an option. We decided to have the funeral on Friday. Every night until then, I was not going to sleep until I saw the first trace of sunlight. My friends could not convince me to do otherwise, so they joined me in my crazy quest. For five nights, Trena, Shelly, and her family stayed on the phone with me through the wee hours. We talked and laughed. One night, we played an impromptu game of Bible trivia. Shelly always stayed up the longest. Her voice was the last I heard as the sun began to shine through Cole's room window. My friends stepped in the face of my fear with me. They helped me battle every night with so much fun that the hours quickly passed.

I managed to get about two to three hours of sleep every morning until Thursday. This was Cole's day to say goodbye. Lieber Correctional approved the request for him to attend Granddaddy's funeral. Once again, Aunt Barbara had a different idea. This one turned out to be very good. We held a private viewing for Cole on Thursday afternoon before the wake that evening. It would be held at the funeral home. We let a select group of family members know about this private viewing. This avoided nosy eyes and potential confrontation. Cole needed to be surrounded only by people whose love he did not question.

Thursday afternoon, I anxiously stood outside the funeral home doors, waiting for my brother. We had not seen each other in months and I missed him. The unmarked van pulled up into the reserved parking space closest to the door. Uniformed, South Carolina Department of Correction Officers got out. Both had guns in waist holsters. One met the other on the passenger side to open the back door. Cole's shackled feet stepped down before I saw his face. The officers said something to him. One stood on each side, walking him to the funeral home entrance. We were instructed not to make physical contact with him during the viewing, meaning I could not hug my brother.

We went inside to the aunts and cousins waiting for him, along with my mother. He greeted everyone before going into the chapel. Cole sat on the front pew to see Granddaddy's body lay in the black casket. I watched from the lobby. Tears wet my brother's face. He looked over and motioned me to come but that was not going to happen. I had no desire to see death's image again until absolutely necessary.

After a while, he came out of the chapel. Family members brought plates of collard greens, baked macaroni, and cake for him. The Correction Officers were kind. They allowed him to eat and take some food for the road as long as he shared. Cole talked and caught up with everyone. The allotted two hours went by fast. Everyone walked to the door as he was escorted back to the van. The officers helped his shackled feet up the step. He lifted his cuffed wrists to wave once more before they closed the doors. The humid Charleston heat could not pierce the somberness as we watched the van pull off.

The next day, I had to see the image for the last time. The face looked much closer to the grandfather I knew. The life was gone though, which made it easier to accept Granddaddy was not there. The rest of the family walked by. Finally, in front of a packed church, Sandra and Barbara stood at their father's casket. My aunt's cries were audible but my mother's were not. She just stood. Aunt

Barbara tried to lead her back to the pew, but she would not move. She pulled her arm away from her big sister. My mother, Sandra Smalls, took the overlays and gently laid them, one by one, over her Daddy's face. Then, she reached her tiny hand up to close the casket cover. Finally, she turned around to face her seat. She slowly walked back with the residual limp from the accident.

The deep sadness on my mother's face was heartbreaking. For the last year, her Daddy was the one familiar person in her life. She may have recognized family members and old friends, but they were different from what she remembered. Her Daddy's unchanged presence was comforting for her. The stability she depended on was gone. Her childhood home was the only familiar aspect of her life but all that was about to change. In a few days, she would be living in a house she did not remember, with a daughter she did not know. I realized her sadness was mixed with fear. But then, the only fear I felt was my own.

Getting New Wheels

Thirty days after we buried Granddaddy, Mr. Brickman called the four daughters to his office for the reading of Granddaddy's will. He also called Auntie Mina. I rode in the car with my mother and Aunt Barbara. Aunt Debbie and Aunt Nana came separately. Lines were drawn. The will revealed Auntie Mina would oversee those lines and everything else. Granddaddy appointed her as personal executor of his estate. She possessed authority to settle any disputes over his property and assets not covered in the will. Disputes came quickly over things like money in bank accounts and his truck. There was one asset on which they were all able to agree. I would continue to drive the white Chrysler LeBaron.

Now more than ever, I hated that car. I should have been in the office to tell them I did not want it. Instead, I sat in that car waiting for them to come out. Another decision was made about my life without my input. Aunt Debbie said they felt it would be unfair to take the car from me since I drove it for the last year. I should have been grateful, but I was pissed. My Mama's Buick still sat in Granddaddy's yard, stalled. No one cared about it. The idea of simply recharging the car to allow it to operate at full potential never occurred to them. They were more concerned about the vehicle with more obvious value. They planned to sell Granddaddy's big, red truck and split the money amongst the four sisters. I took the LeBaron to Mama's house when we moved back in.

My mother and I returned to our house the Sunday after the funeral. The transition was difficult. She woke up every night, pacing the halls the same way she did when she had a seizure, but with different intent. My mother would come to my room and stand in the doorway, watching me. There were nights I woke up to her standing over my bed. My eyes opened, she stared into them for a few seconds, then slowly went back to her room. I learned her sleep pattern and began staying up until she awakened in the middle of the night.

Linda was still coming to prepare her for independent living. I planned to leave for college in August. Though her therapy was scheduled to end in June, I was concerned about my mother after Granddaddy's passing. Linda came by for an emergency visit the day after he died. I told her about the plan to return to Mama's house following the funeral. She graciously decided to continue weekly visits for one more month to help my mother settle into her new home. Linda observed meal prep, laundry, and household tasks. She also helped with resources outside the home like grocery delivery services and alternative transportation options for doctor visits. Her last visit was bittersweet. She was happy with the enormous progress my mother made since their first meeting and was confident in her ability to live on her own. I understood her job was over but I was truly sad to see her go.

I wanted to be as confident as Linda, but it was hard. Watching my mother navigate typical adult tasks was like giving a sixteen-year-old girl the key to the house for the weekend. Though cognitively capable of doing basic things, she could not necessarily handle the responsibility on her own. I tried to get my mother accustomed to properly using the services Linda introduced. She made grocery lists for the store to deliver but the items tended to be duplicates of what she already had in the cabinet. I went with her in the Dial-A-Ride van to the doctor but I called to schedule the ride. Otherwise, she would miss the three-day deadline. Time was running out and so was my sanity.

I thought finally being home would make me feel better about everything that happened over the past year, but it was wishful thinking. As my mother settled into the house, the place felt less and less like home. I was uncomfortable all the time. Stress and staying up at night took a toll on my menstrual cycle. Months went by without a flow. Large sections of my hair fell out. The back part of my head was bald from my ear to the nape of my neck. Nothing was the same or anywhere close to how I pictured life would return for me. I was scared. Even if it was just a small piece of my dreams, I needed to hold on to it. Going away to college was urgent.

After the fourth of July, I tried to shift my mind to college preparations. The first order of business was getting rid of the LeBaron. While I hated that car, it was also not practical for school. Major mechanical issues plagued the Chrysler which did not allow it to make the three-hour road trips back and forth to UNC Charlotte. I figured the best option would be to sell it and use the money to get Mama's old Buick up and running again. A new battery and insurance were all it needed. But selling the LeBaron would have to go through Aunt Barbara because I was still a minor. The little bullet point about me in the lawyer's office was settled but the actual legal documents said the car belonged to my mother. Aunt Barbara handled my mother's money since Granddaddy's death, though my mother could still write checks. I talked to my aunt about the idea of selling the LeBaron and she was firmly against it. She was even more against the idea of me going away to college. Her solution was selling Mama's car instead. We would get more for it because it was a later model. As for college, she could not believe I still considered going away to a university. She made it known months earlier while watching me fill out registration materials. Trident Technical College seemed like the best option to her. Then, I would get a "nice, little job" and stay in Charleston to take care of my mother. Everything she said made logical sense for an ordinary person on Liberty Hill destined to stay there. That was not me. I wanted out.

Aunt Barbara's sensible suggestions angered me. They felt like more proof that no one could see me. All people saw was what I did for them and the family. I lost my Mama. My senior year was spent taking care of a woman who barely recognized me. I gave up on my dream of going to bigger universities much farther away and I was told to give up on going to a university altogether. The best I could hope for was community college. I was told to stop dreaming but it was not possible. Everything inside me refused to accept my current situation as a permanent reality.

I was getting rid of that LeBaron, one way or another. There were ways around Aunt Barbara. I decided if she would not help me get Mama's car running then I would get a new car. Trading the LeBaron did not require my Aunt's signature but would require my mother's presence. So, I drove my mother to the big Honda dealership on Rivers Ave. I intended to drive off the lot with a new Honda Civic on a new road to get my future back. After 30 minutes and a test drive, I picked out a car and sat in the dealer's office. Warnings came while we waited for the salesman to return with my mother's credit check. The excitement of buying a new car wore off and I felt how wrong the decision was. The salesman returned to inform us we weren't approved for a brand new car but could still get a used one. He showed us a Mazda Protégé, less than a year old, and it was fine with me. All that mattered was not driving the LeBaron ever again. We went back to the office while he started the paperwork. My mother sat across from me on the other side of the small round table. I searched for the happy and proud look I saw on Mama's face when she bought me the Hyundai more than a year and a half ago, but it wasn't there. What I saw in her face was indifference.

The man came back and told us he managed to get the dealership to give $1,000 for the LeBaron. This would serve as part of the down payment. They would need another $500 more to get the monthly payments down to what we could afford. It felt like I was somehow being taken for a ride, but I did not care. I asked my mother to write the check. She gave it to the salesman who immediately paused.

"Who's Barbara Doctor?"

My heart sank. I knew she replaced Granddaddy's name on my mother's checks but didn't think it would be a problem. I was able to use them for my senior supplies a few months back. There was never an issue.

"She's my sister," my mother replied.

"Hmm," the salesman said. "To be on the safe side, I'm going to have to at least call to keep things on the up and up. Do you have her number?"

"Yeah," my mother said as she wrote the number down.

That was it. I knew once he called Aunt Barbara, this whole thing would be over. A dreaded lecture was certain. My teenage brain thought about my friends, and how I told them I was getting a new car. The embarrassment sunk in just as the man came back to his office.

"OK. We're all set."

I was confused. "Did you talk to her," I asked?

"Yes, she had a few questions, understandably. But she said everything's OK."

I was shocked and a bit suspicious. There was no way I expected her to allow this to happen when she had the power to stop it. What was her angle? I decided to table my suspicions as my mother signed the papers and I handed the LeBaron keys over to the salesman. Giving him those keys felt better than receiving the ones to the new car. The happiness was not what I imagined but at least I was driving something that felt close to being mine. I knew I would still have to call Aunt Barbara when we got back to the house.

The call was short. She didn't say much. I explained my reasons for getting the car and all the financials. I planned to make the monthly payments with the child support checks from my biological father. When she asked about insurance, I told her we would get some that day. To pay for it, I would get a job at school. Aunt Barbara provided the name of the insurance company for the LeBaron and said to just transfer the policy to the new car. She gave a very stern warning about the financial responsibilities of the car. My aunt had serious doubts that I would be able to maintain it. But she did not fuss. There was no lecture. She said what she had to say and let it go. I was relieved. Like her, I also had doubts but I chose to let it go.

There were two features the Mazda came with, which I sorely missed while driving the LeBaron: air-conditioning and a tape deck. The blazing, humid heat of Charleston summers might kill a person in a car without an air conditioner. Being able to eliminate the scorching car torture was worth any lecture. Being able to listen to my treasured cassette tapes was another welcomed change. Both features came in handy during the drive to UNC Charlotte for an orientation. The trip was two days and included a test to determine my eligibility for certain courses. Tours of a few class buildings were also available. I wanted to take the chance to get familiar with the city again. My last time here was the spring break before Mama's accident. This would be my first trip to the school by myself. It would also be my mother's first night alone in the house. The trip provided a good barometer for how both of us would handle our new surroundings.

I made sure everything was set for my mother. Aunt Barbara knew when I was leaving and when to expect me on the next day. As I got on the road Friday afternoon, I thought about the last time I made this trip. The vision of my Mama standing in the open doorway was etched in my brain. I had to shake it. I put in my Raphael Saadiq cassette tape and began to blast his voice singing *Ask of You*. The song quickly made me think of David. Before I knew it, I arrived in Charlotte, NC. I checked into the Holiday Inn and asked for directions to the nearest mall. Tons of job opportunities would be available there. After checking out the stores, I went to a Wal-Mart near the hotel, bought some dinner, and finally settled in for the evening.

The next day started very early. Orientation was at 8:00 a.m. Still unfamiliar with the campus, I wanted to arrive in time to look for the building. The day went rather quickly after finding it. I took the test and sat through orientation. Everything was done by 11:00 a.m. I went back to the mall to pick up a dress I saw for Shelly before getting on the road. Again, my mind drifted to Mama. It would be so different if she was here. Mama would have a ton of questions about the test and orientation. I wondered if we would have been in a good enough place to enjoy the trip without arguing. Just the thought of her tongue lashing was enough to make me grateful I made the trip alone. Then, I remembered the woman who was waiting in Mama's house.

While I was confident my mother could make it through one night by herself, I still hoped she was okay. She sat, watching television in the den when I returned in the afternoon. Things went smoothly while I was gone. The house had not burned down from any meals she prepared over the last twenty-four hours. She took all her medicine as scheduled. Quietly standing at the door, I was relieved, yet let down. There was no concern coming out of the room, only cigarette smoke. My mother didn't ask how my trip went or if I was excited about going to college. She never looked up to say hello. I wanted her to care but it seemed like she didn't. Turning to my bedroom, I walked in and quickly unpacked, looking for the dress bought for Shelly. I grabbed the clothing store bag and left for my friend's house.

The connection between Shelly and I got stronger over the summer after graduation when Trena went to visit her family in Florida. Hours at Shelly's house were part of my daily routine. We talked about boys, our family problems, and the future. Other days, we watched the same movies or listened to the same music over and over. We critiqued artists and made predictions about their careers. All day long, we were together.

Though our friendship felt like medicine for my sanity, it was more like the liquor I drank to numb my pain. Long periods with Shelly occasionally led to my bad decisions. I should have recognized it the week before I left for UNC Charlotte. On Sunday night, I was driving the Mazda with Shelly in the passenger seat. We decided to go by Illusions, the teen nightclub. Many of our friends were there, but we were looking for the guy Shelly liked. We just wanted to drive by and see who was outside. I slowed the car as we approached the front of Illusions.

"Do you see anybody?" I asked. My eyes were straight ahead.

"No, just hold up," she said. "Slow down a little bit more."

I slowed the car down to almost a crawl.

"Ooh," Shelly said with excitement. She obviously saw someone. I wanted to see, too.

"What?" I shouted.

I turned my head to the passenger side window. It wasn't more than a few seconds before we felt the crash. I looked forward and saw the smashed military license plates of a white van. Its reverse lights were still on. When I turned my head to see what Shelly was looking at, I also turned the steering wheel, taking the car off the road and into a parking lot next to the teen club.

My heart raced as we got out of the car. We had no injuries. Neither did the van's passenger and driver. We exchanged information. I was still shaking when I saw a friend from North Charleston High approaching. Ironically, it was the same guy Shelly was trying to see. I didn't have the energy for jokes or nosy questions. My sharp tongue was ready until I saw the genuine concern in his eyes.

"Call my daddy," he said calmly.

His father owned Action Auto Body Shop. I made the call and waited for the tow truck. Shelly stood next to me as I watched the Mazda being lifted onto the truck bed. It had been less than a month since I told my aunt about the car. Now, I had to tell her I wrecked it. She was right. How was I going to get to college? How was I going to get off The Hill? My dreams were crushed and sitting on the back of a tow truck.

"It's totaled," I said, looking at the car.

I was about to fall apart in the middle street. As I began to sink, I felt Shelly's arm around mine.

"No, it's not," she said firmly. "It can be fixed."

She held me up. A few minutes later, her sister came and took me to my house.

I was so relieved to see Willie at the kitchen table with my mother. Having him there took some of the pressure off of making the call to Aunt Barbara. Her response was similar to when I bought the car. She did not scold me as expected. My aunt was calm and practical about the situation. She asked if I was okay and told me to call the insurance company in the morning. I went to my room after we hung up. Aunt Barbara could have said, "I told you so" but she didn't. I almost wished she did because I felt like an irresponsible idiot. The LeBaron was gone. I wrecked the Mazda, and Mama's car sat stalled in Granddaddy's yard. Fear gripped me as I sat on the bed. I was stuck and there was no one to blame but me.

The Ol' College Try

S helly was right. The car was not totaled. The people at Action Auto Body lived up to their name. They immediately began work on the car intending to finish by Labor Day. Aunt Barbara surprised me when she said her son, Terry, would take me to school in Granddaddy's red truck. I didn't expect her to help me. She was so adamant about me staying home. I wasn't sure a home existed for me anymore. Mama's house was in some weird limbo and I was blocking its transition. The weight of those feelings was heavy. I felt getting out of the house would free me from it, so I spent the last night before leaving, at Shelly's house. As her sister drove me back early the next morning, I knew I did something wrong. Being with friends on my last night, instead of my mother, was selfish.

The guilt ate at me when I walked through the door. My mother sat at the kitchen table as I packed the last few items. By the time Terry arrived, my guilt was swallowed by pain. I always imagined Mama with me on my first day of college. She would make my room up and probably nag about something. Willie and maybe Cole would try to calm her down. They would move the big trunk and lift boxes. There would be lots of smiles and chatter but today was different. My cousin took me to school with my mother. They helped me unpack. Terry was very helpful with the heavy stuff. He even got me to smile a few times.

On the other side of the dorm room, my roommate had settled in earlier. Her bed was made, and CDs were stacked. Terry scanned them to determine if she was white. We assumed she was, after seeing several country music titles and her name. My mother and Terry were a little concerned about me living with a white girl but I didn't care so much. I was very comfortable around white people.

Liberty Hill allowed generations of residents to convince themselves the only people who can be trusted were people like them. When I crossed the railroad tracks, I learned something different. I hated Buist Academy but going there allowed me to experience great friendships with girls who looked nothing like me. Having this roommate would allow me to finally have the sleepover the culture did not permit when I was a little girl.

Terry and my mother went with me to find one of my classes. For a minute, I thought my mother was proud of me. Her eyes were a little brighter as we passed through campus. We walked back to the dorms, hugged goodbye, and they headed back to Charleston. I went up to the dorm room and waited to meet my roommate.

Polly didn't come in until later that evening. She was at work. A few weeks before the semester started, she managed to come to Charlotte and secure a job at a fast-food restaurant. She worked full-time hours until classes started. Her job was a necessity as she was paying for her truck and putting herself through school. I felt so behind the curve. I didn't think of applying for a position when I went to those mall stores during my orientation trip. Meeting Polly and watching her independence gave me a new drive. I wanted to catch up with her. The Friday before Labor Day, I caught a Greyhound bus to North Charleston to get the car. I was going to drive back to Charlotte, get a job and work my way through school.

Without my car, I was forced to stay on campus. I managed to meet a few people who were great to be around. The first night, I met one girl by simply leaving my dorm room door open. She happened to be in my chemistry class, and we started walking together. We met other girls who joined our walks to the science building. I enjoyed walking with them, particularly Janiece. She had a sophisticated maturity I admired. We often made plans to hang out and study together. As the semester went by, I was a repeated no-show. Every day, I debated going to class. Instead of sitting in Chemistry or Algebra, I sat in my dorm room watching soap operas and music videos. I tried looking for a job but gave up when I didn't hear from the stores where I applied. I was somewhat relieved because it meant my weekends were free to drive to Charleston. I desperately missed Shelly and Trena. I also missed David.

I thought about David every day from the moment I set foot on campus. Thinking about him was one of the few things that helped get my mind off my mother. I would sometimes be consumed with worry about her being in the house alone. My heart slowly filled with guilt for going to college and resentment followed closely. It was like a painful, never-ending roller coaster of emotions I could not control. Letting my mind drift to David was the distraction I used to calm my nerves. We had not seen each other since prom weekend. I wondered how he was doing. I wondered if he was adjusting to college life better than I was.

In my desk drawer was a letter I wrote to David over the summer but never sent. My feelings for him were handwritten on beautifully colored stationary. I admitted my fear of actually saying the written words because my heart was already so fragile the past year. Before sealing the letter, I read it over and over. I took it with me to Charlotte, hoping I would get up enough nerve to send it to him. After a few weeks into the semester, I was ready to mail the letter but we had not exchanged our college addresses. He was attending one of the universities in Charleston, but his pager number was all I had, which was a long-distance number. My best friends came in handy for this situation.

Shelly started her senior year at North Charleston High in August. She knew I needed to talk to David, so she took matters into her own hands and paged him. He recognized the number as one from which I often paged him and called back immediately. When Shelly answered, she explained the long-distance situation and got his phone number for me. She gave me his number and said he was waiting for my call. I could not hide behind excuses anymore. It took several minutes but I finally dialed the number. His roommate answered and told me I had just missed him. My heart sank. I waited too long. But just before accepting defeat, his roommate asked to take a message.

"Just tell him Ruthenna called," I said.

"Oh, hold on. He's been waiting for you. Don't hang up."

My hand was almost shaking while I held the phone. After a few seconds, I heard his voice.

"Hello?"

I lit up. "Hey. How are you?

I hoped he didn't hear me blushing. We jumped into a lengthy catch-up conversation. He was so happy I decided to go to UNC Charlotte. David was concerned about me since prom night. He knew I was struggling and was afraid I would give up on who I could be. I tried to reassure him that was not going to happen. Unfortunately, I was not so confident. I quickly changed the subject to our class schedules and roommate stories. We talked a bit more before noticing the late hour. He insisted I call him the next time I came home. I agreed but, in the meantime, we would write each other. This was my chance.

"I have something I've been meaning to send you anyway."

"For real?" he asked curiously.

"Yeah. You asked for one of my senior pictures a long time ago. Remember?"

"That's right," he recalled. "You tried to give me one without writing anything on the back."

"I know. Well, I finally wrote something."

I didn't tell him about the letter. The plan was to simply slip it into the box with the framed picture he wanted. I told him to expect the package soon. We said good night and hung up.

The next day, I sent the letter. Weeks passed and I heard nothing from David. I didn't know what to think. Was the letter too much? Did I scare him? What if it got lost in the mail? Maybe he never received it. I was getting frustrated with not hearing from him and vented to Shelly. She suggested I just call him when I came home the next weekend, but I didn't want to do it. My heart was poured out in that letter. The least he could do was let me know he received it. Shelly reminded me that David never left me in the dark. She believed there was some explanation for why I hadn't heard from him. If I wanted the truth, I would have to reach out.

I took her advice the next weekend and paged him on Sunday evening. He surprised me by calling back because the number was not familiar. I was avoiding going back to my mother's and decided to spend the last night in town, with my oldest sister, Tee. David somehow knew to ask for me when she answered. I picked up the phone in the kitchen and sat down. Too nervous to go right to the letter, I made small talk but we knew the conversation was pointless. During an awkward silence, I dove in.

"Did you get my letter?"

"Yeah, I got it," he answered.

"So," I said. "Questions? Comments? Concerns?"

"Oh, I think that's something we need to talk about face to face. Right?"

I was caught off guard and could not respond.

"Hello?" he checked.

"Yeah," I answered. "I'm here."

"Well, maybe you should be here," David retorted. "If I give you directions, can you come over?"

"Yeah. Um. Just let me get a pen."

I quickly found a pen and took the directions. He wanted to meet somewhere for food before showing me to the university guest parking. I agreed to meet him.

So many things ran through my mind while driving down Interstate 26. Many thoughts were about God. The second I hung up the phone from David, I knew what would happen on this visit and I wanted Him to see it. He saw the very tumultuous weekend I had. My mother violently blew up at me during one of her episodes on my first night. Did He see it? I ended up at Shelly and Trena's house where I unintentionally used them as an outlet for the anger I couldn't unleash on my mother. We had a huge argument causing me to storm out of their home too. Did He see that? Did He see me driving around in the Mazda for the last two days, because it was the only place where I felt comfortable? By Sunday, I was able to resolve things with Shelly and Trena, but I was still very angry. The weekend reminded me of the harsh reality of my life. My friends were grossly inaccurate targets of the anger I should have aimed directly at God. David was the ultimate arrow. For years, I pushed him away because I loved God more. I trusted Him and his plan for my life. Without question, I sacrificed so much believing He knew what was best for me. Tonight, I had a whole lot of questions, but I was not in the mood for His answers. I was in the mood for payback.

I saw David waiting for me when I pulled into the parking lot. He, charmingly, opened my door.

"Hey," he said as we immediately embraced.

All of my anger and anxiety from the weekend faded into the background. I settled into the sincere arms of someone who wanted nothing but to hold me. We were silent for a bit. He still held my hand when we pulled away.

"You wanna get something to eat?" he asked.

"No," I answered. "I'm not really hungry."

He got a little snack and we headed to his dorm. The resident advisor at the front desk was a bit hesitant to let me up because curfew was quickly approaching. David explained I was from out of town. I showed him my UNC Charlotte identification and he was very understanding. He reminded David that visitors had to leave in about an hour, but he was willing to let me stay a little longer. We thanked him and went upstairs. We were still joking about the situation when we got off the elevator. I heard the TV as he took out his keys to open the door.

"Oh, your roommate's home?" I asked.

179

"Nah, he went to the Million Man March," he replied.

"Really," I said. "They had a meeting in my dorm about that. A whole busload of guys from my school are going." We walked into his room.

"Yeah, they're taking some buses from here too," he said while setting my things down. "My roommate helped plan the trip." David went over to his dresser and picked up a stack of CDs.

"Ugh," he sighed. "He took all the good music with him." He settled on an old SWV album.

His dorm room was a little smaller than mine. We talked about dorm life. He enjoyed rooming with his best friend. I laughed at the idea of having Shelly as a roommate.

"We would probably kill each other," I told him. "We're too much alike."

He laughed. I sat on his bed next to where he lay, and he asked me how school was going. The truth was it was not going well. I hated it. I felt out of place. I wasn't putting much effort into my classes. No one cared about my performance in high school, but this was worse because I didn't care. I did not want David to know I was losing all motivation. I couldn't tell him I was lost. Instead, I told him a new plan I concocted.

"I'm leaving after this semester."

He looked at me, stunned. "What?! You gonna drop out of school?" His tone changed quickly to shock and disappointment. I had to say something to ease his concern.

"I'm not dropping out," I said. "I'm just gonna wait out next semester." I started making things up as I went along. David's eyes squinted with doubt.

"I know they say most people don't go back when they drop out but that's not me. I'm going back. I'm just gonna transfer to a different school."

"Where?" he asked.

"Maybe somewhere in Georgia or even Chapel Hill. Shelly, Trena, and I want to go to the same school. I'm waiting to see where Shelly gets recruited. She's getting a lot of track scholarship offers." It sounded good in my head.

"You just said you couldn't live with her," he argued.

I was getting frazzled. "We don't have to room together. She'll probably be in some kind of athletic housing, anyway. You know how athletes get special treatment." He was quiet. "I'll go back to school, David. It'll work out."

He still would not say anything, and I felt his frustration. I had to distract him.

"Could you mute the TV or something?" I asked. "The music and the television are too much."

He turned the TV off. His arm slowly fell in my lap as he laid down. I knew he didn't believe a word I was saying. I didn't either, but I didn't care.

Listening to me talk about my future was sad. I was losing sight of who I was and who I wanted to be. It frightened and angered me. David was talking but I couldn't hear him over my fear. I grabbed his hand to calm me as it had done so many times in the past. Holding his hand was not working. I needed more. He stopped talking when I looked deep into his eyes. Finally, I said the hell with it. I leaned down and kissed him. The kiss was soft but aggressive. I stopped for a moment with my head against his. Taking a breath, I kissed him again.

David and I had several passionate encounters throughout high school. He was always gentle and caring with me. Each encounter took us closer and closer to the point of no return, but I always stopped him. I was committed to God with the most intimate part of myself. Now, I felt our commitment was broken. God hurt me. Events of the past year flashed under my eyelids as I allowed every kiss to grow hotter and deeper. Suddenly, David pulled back, trying to read my face. He knew something was different about me this time.

"Are you sure?" he whispered.

His genuine concern made me want this even more. I lifted his shirt off his chest.

"I'm sure."

He was still reluctant. I knew he would not go further if I did not lead. Softly, I kissed the muscles on his abdomen and up to his neck. We faced each other and he gently kissed me once more.

"Tell me if you want me to stop."

I nodded. Tonight, there were no plans of stopping.

When I was younger, Mama told me the first time I had sex would be painful, but I did not feel pain tonight. As David laid me down on the bed, my mind drifted in and out. I thought about the plan I explained earlier. Seeing myself walking around on a campus I dreamed about before Mama's accident was soothing.

"Pleasure is the destination," SWV sang softly on the CD player. I heard the song before, but the slow beat was unfamiliar. It was nice, bringing me back into the room with David's lips on spots they never touched. My body shifted and my mind went to the three-hour drive I had to make the next day. This life was not a dream. Reality sank in and so did David; slowly, over and over. The sensation of his body inside mine was not satisfying. I wanted my dream back.

"Stop," I whispered. "Just stop."

David looked into my eyes. He knew I didn't want this anymore. After touching one side of my face and softly kissing the other, he sat up.

We did not speak one word as we got dressed. He helped me with my jacket and walked me out the door. The act, I knew would hurt God the most, was done. I wanted to feel vindicated, but I only felt numb. David watched me on the elevator.

"Are you alright?" he asked.

"Yeah," I said. "I'm fine."

He was still looking at me when the doors opened. We walked to my car and stood at the door in silence. I didn't look at him.

"You sure you're okay?"

"Yeah, I'm just thinking about this long drive ahead of me," I said.

"You're not driving back tonight, are you?"

"No, no. I'll get on the road in the morning." I could tell he was relieved.

"Well, call me. Let me know you got to Charlotte safe."

"I will."

He took me in his arms and held me close. I wanted to stay in that embrace, but we had to let go.

I was glad I gave myself to David. There was no one on the planet I wanted to be with that way, except my husband. Marriage was the original plan. College was the original plan too, but the plan was going up in smoke. My virginity was the one thing I could control. It was mine to keep and mine to give away. I chose when to give it and who received it. My only hope was that He was watching.

I headed straight to Shelly's house when I left David.

"Shelly. Room. Now," I yelled as I rushed past her and her sisters at the kitchen table.

Smiling widely, Shelly quickly got up and followed me to her room. I gave her a full recap of the evening. She listened and asked questions. Nothing was off-limits. The conversation was no different from all the other intimate conversations we could not have with anyone else.

After the night with David, I stayed at Shelly's house until Tuesday. Going to Charleston on Fridays after Chemistry class was a bad habit I developed. My intention was always to get back on the road by 9:00 a.m. Monday, to be back in time for Chemistry by 1:00 p.m. The problem was Sunday nights. Shelly and I would stay up talking all night at her house. Going to school was still mandatory for her. She had to go, regardless of how tired she was. College students don't have the same pressure. So, I ignored the responsibility by saying I was too tired to drive. Textbooks went home with me which was pointless since I never opened them. The number of missed assignments was growing. My test grades were horrible. Subjects that should have been easy were unnecessary struggles. I tried to justify my choices with excuses. The class was so large, no one missed me. I avoided walking through campus for fear of seeing other students I met when I first arrived. The notion that people did not notice my absence was false. Janiece noticed and she was very concerned.

Janiece and I shared a Drama class on Monday night and my presence there was scarce as well. She knew I went home every weekend. I told her about my friends and how much I missed them. I made my trips seem like the most fun. She was skeptical and I felt I had something to prove. I invited her with me for a weekend. Though she had a good time, she did not see what made me make the three-hour drive every Friday. It was not worth the sacrifice to her. She saw more in me and made me aware others saw it too.

Our Drama teacher noticed my absence. I was one of the few active participants in the room of fifty students and the professor had highlighted my work. Janiece told me he was quite aware when I was missing. Finally, he confronted me about it on a night I decided to show up. He pulled me aside before class.

"I just wanted to check in with you, Ruthenna."

I didn't realize he knew my name. My heart was beating so fast. I felt like a rat caught when the lights turned on.

"Is everything ok?" he asked.

"Oh yes, everything's fine," I replied.

"Are you sure? You started so well. Now I rarely see you."

I didn't argue the point, but I tried to cover it up. "I know. It's just…I have to go home on the weekends. My mother is sick and I have to check-in." This was such a load of crap but I played it.

"Ok. I just hate to see you fail this class. You have so much promise and it's clear this is something you enjoy."

I was getting close to tears. Having someone believe in me was difficult to swallow. I didn't know why.

"No, you're right," I said. "This is the only class I look forward to."

"I look forward to you being here. The whole class does." Every word he said made me feel more sorry for myself. I wanted the conversation to be over. I nodded my head.

"Ok, well if there's anything I can do, please, let me know. I want you to succeed here."

"I will. Thank you."

I followed him back into the classroom knowing I needed to make some serious changes. That conversation should have been a turning point in my college career, but it wasn't. The professor's faith in me was one voice among countless others in my head screaming doubt and fear.

The weekend trips continued to the end of the semester. I completely gave up by Thanksgiving. Trying to catch up in my classes was a cumbersome task. I barely passed Drama and failed the math course. I didn't bother to turn in the last paper in my English class. The Chemistry final exam was pointless after not attending a full week of class in months. I hated myself for not being motivated. On a cold Saturday morning in mid-December, I packed up my dorm room. Confusion emerged as I looked at the tall, high-rise once more before getting into the car. There was no doubt I was leaving someplace I was meant to be but leaving felt right too. I shook my head and got into the Mazda, headed back to Liberty Hill.

A Bad Reunion

A nd I'm supposed to love you. But I don't know you either."
I heard the line from the television as if it were directed
at me, yet it wasn't. A beloved character on General
Hospital woke up from a car accident with no memory of his family
or life before the crash. Two months after dropping out of school in
December, I sat in the den on Gaynor Ave., watching this soap opera
and living it. Like the character on the show, Sandra Smalls
Porterfield emerged from her accident a different person. By 1996,
everyone was forced to adjust.

Living with my mother was not scary anymore, but it was still
very strange. I couldn't get used to seeing what seemed like a
fragment of Mama's body, walking around the house. My mother,
Sandra, fit at her childhood home. Here, she looked out of place. I
knew she felt the same way during those first three months at the
house. Her feelings changed while I was in North Carolina. She
made the house her own. Little things were rearranged like china in
Mama's beautifully decorated dining room. Bedroom linens were
mismatched. Changes were drastic as time passed. She started
throwing things out like shoes, clothes, and decorative pieces. One
day, I saw her wedding album from her first marriage, in the outside
garbage. I asked her why she threw out something she kept for nearly
thirty years.

"What do I need it for," she asked?
The blank look on her face told me she did not care about the events
in that photo album. I wanted to say, "For me." Mama planned to
save her wedding dress and the photo album for my future. This
meant nothing to the woman sitting in front of me. I couldn't say
anything. The memories were gone. The album was hers to do with
what she wanted.

All pictures and mementos were in danger of being thrown out. Sometimes she removed photos from albums or frames, only keeping pictures of people she remembered. A cube frame that once held six snapshots only held one picture of her Daddy. I never found the pictures of me or my siblings. My heart sank as I watched my Mama's life being erased from her home. The only way to deal with the changes was by reminding myself they weren't mine. Though my life was a part of her memories, the items she discarded were hers. It wasn't long before she crossed the line. The day I saw my Miss WPAL trophy moved to the living room; I was annoyed. Being grateful not to find it in the trash, I did not say anything.

My mother's daily routine included meals, cleaning, and television. Living independently was not a challenge anymore but managing episodes was still an issue. Aunt Barbara was an indirect target of her outbursts while I was gone. My aunt experienced small doses of what I went through at Granddaddy's house, however, she had the luxury of going back to her own home. My return put me right back in the line of fire.

Returning from college broke my mother's routine of living alone. When I was in the kitchen or walking the hall, the new sounds were triggers leading to episodes different from the ones before I left. My mother developed a huge level of paranoia. She believed the pots and pans in the cabinets did not belong to her. People were taking her towels and dishes and replacing them with ones from her Daddy's house. I often caught her trying to remove the thermostat console from the wall because she believed someone changed it. Trying to explain things to her was like talking to a brick wall. The only solution was to calm her down enough to go back in the den and watch TV. Sometimes it worked, and other times her paranoia would be coupled with violence. One day she broke my bedroom door off the hinges, swearing she heard me singing the music playing through my headphones. My mother yanked the cords at my neck and nearly choked me with the headphones. I wondered if the episodes were this severe because I was doing something wrong or because Granddaddy was no longer there to curb them. Either way, I could not handle this. I had to address the violent behavior at her next doctor's appointment.

A different doctor walked in the exam room every time, always in a white lab coat. They would read her chart and do basic exams. Some of them were nice and personable. Others were cold. This time, I hoped to get an empathetic one. A tall, white man with dark hair walked in, flipping through papers on his clipboard. This doctor asked a few questions, glancing at my mother once before taking out his stethoscope for the usual exam. Then, I asked him a few questions of my own. I explained what was happening. My mother interjected as I was giving him examples of her paranoid episodes. She firmly said someone was replacing her things. Her outburst nearly embarrassed me but then I was grateful. At least he saw what I was talking about. After hearing everything, he asked my mother more questions about how she was feeling. She told him no pain and her last seizure was months ago, before ringing in the new year.

"What about emotionally? Have you felt depressed at all?" the doctor asked.

Something about his tone seemed off. The other physicians usually sat down at this point in the exam. In the corner of the room, sat a vacant metal stool with wheels.

"Depressed?" my mother responded.

"Well, have you felt very sad at times?" he continued, still standing.

My mother looked lost in her thoughts.

"It does get lonely sometimes. You know when you're in a house by yourself. You can't drive anywhere. Sitting in that den. You get tired of watching TV all the time. But whatchu gonna do?"

I felt for her and I knew it must be hard. It did not occur to me how lonely my mother was.

"Hmm," the doctor muttered, turning towards the counter on the wall.

I looked at him, hoping he did not forget about the violent episodes. The physician quickly scribbled something on a pad.

"Ok," he said. "I'm writing you a prescription for Paxil. It's a new antidepressant. It should help with the mood swings."

"What about her epilepsy medicine?" I asked.

"I'm writing that prescription as well," the doctor dismissively said.

Something was off. I felt too intimidated to speak up, not knowing what to ask. He handed the prescription to my mother and walked out of the room.

Though I was a little uneasy, I was hopeful the medicine would help. My mother's behavior changed a few days after taking the new medicine and not for the better. She was angrier and more violent. Paranoid episodes occurred daily. Any attempts to calm her seemed to escalate the situation. Standing at the thermostat, trying to show her nothing changed, resulted in me being pushed into the wall. Disagreeing with her about what happened to the dishes led to threats of me being "fucked up." One night she came in with a metal vacuum pipe attachment and began hitting me with it because the television was too loud. The new medicine was not working. It was making this woman worse and very scary. The morning after being hit with the pipe, I called the hospital, begging them to see my mother as soon as possible. They fit her in the next day.

Once again, a different physician walked into the exam room. Still white but younger, this guy greeted us with a smile before pulling the metal stool from the corner to sit. He looked at her chart and did the same exams as the other doctors.

"I see you were just in last month. What brings you back?"

I explained what happened in the last few weeks. I told him how violent she'd become after starting the new medicine.

"It's not working," I pleaded. "Is there anything else we can try?"

189

The doctor sat silently with wide eyes. "I'm a little concerned for your safety," he said looking at me. "There are options…"

"Oh, no," I quickly interjected. "I'm ok."

He seemed to care more than the last doctor, but I did not want it to lead to extreme measures. Putting my mother away was not an option. While the last few weeks were scary, I assured him I could handle it. I just needed them to fix her medicine. He looked at her chart again. His face changed.

"Paxil?"

"Yes, that's the medicine they put her on," I told him.

He did not look up. He asked a few questions about our last appointment. I told him how I explained her paranoia. I also told him I was not comfortable when the last doctor suggested the new medicine. Then he asked about her epilepsy medication. He was quiet as he carefully read her chart. Finally, he looked up at Mama.

"Well, first let's get you off this medication. Paxil is more for depression patients. It helps regulate moods, but it also increases energy levels. So, if you're already agitated, it could elevate it. That's probably why you were seeing such heightened emotional responses. It also might not be working well with the epilepsy medication."

"So, she can stop taking that new medicine?" I asked.

"Yes, immediately," the doctor answered. "If she was experiencing depressive symptoms, I would say otherwise." He turned to Sandra. "But it sounds like you're just a bit lonely. We need to get you out, around friends and family," he smiled.

I was so relieved, but also angry. My mother was used as a guinea pig. That doctor who prescribed Paxil played with our lives. I wanted to do something but had no idea what. Feeling helpless slowly passed as the young doctor adjusted her epilepsy medications. It decreased the paranoid episodes though they still occurred occasionally. The adjustment to her meds also helped curb

190

her violent reactions. The only remaining problem to solve was her loneliness. I resolved to get her out and around people she loved.

There was one person my mother enjoyed being around. Miss Mable was a quiet and reliable fixture for my family after the accident. She often visited my mother in the hospital. I did not know how much Sandra remembered about Miss Mable, but she was more at ease around her. My mother spent more and more time at Miss Mable's house when we moved out of Granddaddy's. When the doctor said to get her around friends and family, I could think of no one better to trust.

The one thing I happily shared with my mother was the maternal air of Miss Mable's love. She opened the doors of her home to us every day. I drove my mother to her on many mornings. Sometimes, Miss Mable's neighbor or Aunt Barbara would drop her off. They talked, watched TV, and ate Miss Mable's amazing food. She took naps there and occasionally spent the night. The angry episodes did not bother or offend Miss Mable. She knew how to handle them, calming Sandra down in a matter of minutes. Time spent over there significantly helped dissipate her loneliness. My mother always came back from Miss Mable's a little mellower.

When she was home, Sandra continued making the house her own, moving items she did not recognize. The entertainment wall unit in the den was what Mama used as a display for all of my certificates and trophies. The television and other electronics were surrounded from floor to ceiling with years of childhood achievements. Mama had painstakingly set up every award in a decorative manner. Photos attached to some of them. Others matched her gold-plated wine glasses. She often showed the unit to visitors. Mama's pride filled the room when she told people about different medals and awards. I added my high school diploma to the display after graduation. Six months later, I came back to find the unit empty. All that sat in the far right, middle section was the empty cube frame with the photo of Granddaddy inside.

191

"What happened to all my trophies?" I yelled, horrified.

"What are you talking about?" my mother replied.

"What am I talking about? My trophies! My diploma! What did you do with all my stuff?"

"I took all that shit out!" she exclaimed.

"What?!" My heart raced. The image of everything in the trash made me tremble uncontrollably. I ran to the kitchen and checked the trash can and the outside garbage. Nothing was there. I came back to the den.

"Where did you put everything?!" I asked frantically.

"I packed it up and put it in the closet."

I opened the den closet door. A box and some bags sat on the floor. Opening each one, I found everything previously in the unit.

"Oh, my God. No. No." My stomach was in knots. Everything I worked so hard to achieve was packed away like trash.

"Were you seriously going to throw my stuff away?" I asked.

"I can do whatever the fuck I want. This is my house!" she yelled.

"But, this is my stuff!" I forgot how much ownership meant to her. Having authority and marking her territory was vitally important. She constantly reminded me of my place.

"This is my house. You can get the fuck out!" She was triggered. With no strength to deal with an episode, I stood up. Tears were coming.

"I'm asking you. Please. Please, do not throw these things away."

She did not respond. I found some tape to seal the box and pushed the bags to the back of the closet. Maybe, if she didn't see it, they wouldn't be in danger.

I went to my room and sat on the bed, still in shock. The tears fell as I realized there was another fight on my hands. My mother was removing any and everything representing a life she did not know. This woman wanted to erase me. I really needed my Mama. I looked for her in other parts of the house. The living room was the only place remaining with her touch. The walls, the carpet, and the drapery were reminders of the year she remodeled. Vibrant mauve and blue colors evoked solace when I sat on her soft loveseat. In the corner was my Miss WPAL trophy. Mama would never have put one of my greatest achievements there like a yard sale trinket. My mother was making her mark on every part of this house.

Later, in March, I came back one afternoon, to find her sitting on the bed in my room, flipping through my senior year scrapbook. Her eyes were skimming through it like she was at some public display of someone's life. The drawer where I kept the scrapbook was open along with others. Books, programs, and pictures containing personal memories I held very close to my heart were scattered across the carpet floor. It felt like a home invasion.

"What are you doing?" I yelled.

She lifted her head, surprised. I didn't care what she wanted to know or what she was trying to do. She had crossed a boldly defined line in my head.

"This is mine," I declared.

My tone put her on immediate defense. She gave the threatening chuckle I had heard before.

"Humph," she said. "This is my house. I can do whatever I want in my house."

I was so tired of hearing her say it. It made me angrier. She could have every other part of the house, but my room was supposed to be safe. It was supposed to remain untouched by her time capsule memory. The sight of her sitting there with my senior scrapbook was an attack on my memories. My blood was boiling, and I struck back, hard.

"Fine, you wanna know what's in my senior book? I'll read it to you myself."

I took it out of her hands and flipped to the page with entries for the best and worst days of my life. A part of me imagined this happening. Did I hope for it? Angered but slightly hesitant, I read aloud.

"Worst Day of My Life: April 10, 1994. The day my mama died, and I got stuck with a retarded leftover." I looked up. "Is that what you wanted to hear? Are you happy now?"

It was a direct hit but the look on her face was major blowback. She did not cry, at least not in front of me. She put her head down and stood up. I thought she might hit me, but she didn't. She did not say a word. She just walked past me and out of the room. In a flood of conflicting emotions, I collapsed onto the floor. Finally, I was able to say what was eating at my insides for the last two years. But the relief came with immediate and achingly deep regret. I ruthlessly hurt her. Guilt would not allow me to stay in the house.

I made myself scarce after that day. Most mornings, I woke up early, ate breakfast, and left. More nights were spent at Shelly and Trena's house. Aunt Debbie's house was a safe haven too. I was on the run but with no place to hide from reality. Everything was catching up to me and I was too blinded by pain to see it.

Bottom

Aunt Debbie's house was full of love and laughter. Along with Uncle Jerome, her small, three-bedroom house held four teenage daughters, a niece, two nephews. and a grandchild. I passed the time there until Shelly and Trena got out of school. If my cousin, Chanel, was not working, I could count on her to be home with her two-year-old daughter, Erica. When Chanel worked, I was always excited yet nervous about the chance to babysit. Fixing her little girl's hair scared me. Chanel was a budding cosmetologist with the prettiest baby I had ever seen. Erica's hairstyles were always adorable.

Playing with Erica was one of my few joys. The light of her childhood innocence always helped me find a smile in the darkest days. I loved to hear her call my name. Once, after not coming by the house since last week, I walked in the door. Uncle Jerome greeted me when I heard the cutest voice in another room.

"T'ala, T'ala, T'ala, T'ala," the voice yelled. It grew louder and louder as it came closer.

Suddenly, Erica burst into the living room at full speed. My heart melted as she hugged my legs.

"T'ala, T'ala! I missed you! Where you been at?" The answer was most likely with Shelly and Trena.

Weekdays centered around my friends' schedules. Almost every morning, I drove Shelly and Trena to school. In the afternoons, I took them home or to track practice. I took Trena to take her SATs. Shelly's high school romance drama included me as an unnecessary character constantly relaying messages between them. My friends' lives became my life because I did not have one. The attachment was getting stronger and increasingly toxic, particularly with Shelly. The only place I wanted to be was her house. She was the only friend I wanted to talk to. Using our shared experiences and similar struggles, I rationalized my growing dependence on our friendship.

Chanel noticed the attachment early. When she asked where I was going, the answer was always the same. She grew very concerned watching how much time and money I spent on the friendship. There were fast food meals and movie tickets. My gas tank straddled empty consistently. I thought I was a devoted friend, proudly telling Chanel how I planned and paid for Shelly's entire eighteenth surprise birthday party. My cousin was livid. She knew I was dangerously behind on car payments. Spending all this money on my friends and not getting any help in return was ridiculous. I tried to explain how they were lifelines for me, especially Shelly. Her sister styled my hair on so many occasions. The doors of their home were always open.

"Of course they are!" Chanel snapped. "Because your wallet is always open."

She encouraged me to test her theory. Reluctantly, I took her challenge on a weekend when Shelly, her sisters, and I made tentative plans to see a new movie. A blowout fight ensued on the phone when I asked for gas money before leaving. The request caught them off guard. After some yelling and name-calling, that was it. The friendship was over, and I was devastated.

Chanel reminded me about K'Lani and other friends who never took advantage of me. She also made me see what was right in front of me. My cousin was listening willingly just as Shelly did before. The difference was Chanel unapologetically told me what I needed to hear. She wanted me to face my demons. The friendship with Shelly was healthy early on, but it became a crutch. It gave me the help I needed to run away from reality.

The biggest challenge to face was the Mazda. I could not remember the last payment made. Trying to keep insurance on the car, I pawned my beloved flute to pay the premium for one month, but the policy lapsed in March. The finance company was relentless.

Knowing they were coming for the car any day, gave me more reason to stay away from my mother's house. The only contact information they had was hers. They couldn't take the car if they couldn't find me, so I hid at Aunt Debbie's house every night.

In the mornings, I went by my stepfather's apartment. He never lived anyplace for too long. After finding where Willie lived, I stopped by during the day because he worked as a janitor at night. Not allowed to come in, I knocked on the door and waited for his answer. When he heard me, I would go to my car and wait for him to come out. We talked for thirty to forty-five minutes. He might give me money if he had it. Sometimes I took him on an errand or to work. Struggling to keep the car was no secret to him. Willie was supportive but had no advice to offer. Instead, he helped me hide from every tow truck we assumed was coming for me. At first, hearing him come up with exit strategies to evade repossession was fun. I enjoyed seeing him smile when we were quasi-successful.

Something was awkward about it, though. Dodging finance companies was not something I saw growing up. Ownership was a major source of pride and a part of the Smalls family identity on Liberty Hill. They owned various pieces of land throughout the neighborhood. Granddaddy was not rich but he only bought things with cash; from cars to rental property. If he could not own it outright, he didn't buy it. The financial wisdom was passed down to his children.

Aunt Debbie may not have been raised by Granddaddy, but she held the same values. One evening after the insurance lapsed, she talked to me about my finances. Aunt Debbie didn't press me about my situation despite practically moving into her home, however, she was aware of my car troubles without details. The night she called me into her room, she asked about it and I told her how far behind I was. Secretly, I wanted her help but did not want to ask. The last thing I wanted was for her to feel I was taking advantage of her or

LIBERATED FROM THE HILL

that I was a freeloader. After explaining the reasons to keep the car, I waited for her feedback.

"You know, Quala. I know you're responsible. That's why I want to help you. I thought about giving you the money but my problem is what's gonna happen after. Will you be able to keep the car? And what about insurance?"

"No, I know," I replied. "I understand."
She was right. I had no clue how to keep the car. I barely had any idea where I was sleeping from day to day.

Aunt Debbie didn't give me any money that night. Instead, she gave me a reality check. By Easter, losing the car was a certainty. The only question was when. I wanted the answer to be on my terms, but this was getting more difficult by the day. My mother and Aunt Barbara started calling Aunt Debbie, looking for me. A rep from the finance company showed up at my mother's house. He came back the next day, looking for the car. My mother called while he was in front of her for the third time. Chanel sleepily answered the phone early one morning. She held the phone up to the top bunk where I slept. I took the receiver.

"Hello," I nervously said.

"Quala," my mother's voice was unexpectedly calm. "This man here wants to talk to you about this car."

"Ok."

She put the collector on. His firm, authoritative voice came loudly through the phone. He demanded to know where the car was. Fear gripped me. I hung up while he was scolding me about repeatedly having to bother my mother. Then, I passed the phone back down to Chanel.

"Well?" she asked. "What are you gonna do?"

"I don't know."

"Yes, you do know, Quala. Just let the car go. You can't keep running from this."

Chanel was right. She was obviously annoyed too. All the kids went to school, but Erica was still asleep next to her. My issues affected other people. She did not bother to answer when the phone rang again.

"Quala, it's for you."

Climbing down from the top bunk, I reluctantly answered the phone. My mother told me the man left and said he would come back Monday. I had the weekend to bring the car back to the house.

I had to think. Life without the independence I felt only driving provided was unimaginable. Losing the car meant being stuck in my mother's house. I was scared out of my mind until another phone call gave me an idea. A familiar voice came through the receiver. Raquel tracked me down after noticing my absence from church for weeks. She knew I was struggling with life after dropping out of school and decided I needed a break. She invited me on a Florida trip she planned for the teens at Abundant Life and to cover all my expenses. This was my ticket. My sisters moved to Orlando last year after graduation. Giving up the car was not so bad if I knew what happened next. I could go to Florida with Raquel. Call my sisters. Ask to stay with them and start over. I could apply to another university. Get a job. Start fresh. It felt like the perfect solution.

I pulled the car into my mother's driveway on Sunday afternoon and cleared out all of my belongings. After taking the key inside, I headed to my bedroom to pack, stuffing as much as the suitcase could hold. Raquel picked me up a little later. We drove to Florida the next day. The group was smaller than I expected with one church member and her two kids. All five of us shared one hotel room. The trip was way too personal.

The first day after we arrived, a stomach bug kept me from going with everyone on the tours, but I wasn't disappointed. I planned to call my sisters when they departed for Epcot. I figured the number would be listed somewhere. As soon as Raquel and the others left, I flipped through the phone book, searching and searching for

"Porterfield." No luck. I tried to call 411 but was blocked by the hotel switchboard. I tried to think of anyone to call in Charleston who may have their number. Brainstorming led to thoughts of my mother.

The collector would have come for the car by now. Surely, she handed the keys to him without incident, probably happy to have someone stop by. I remembered her talking about her loneliness in the doctor's office. She was lonely when I was there. How bad was the loneliness when she was by herself? I still saw her face when I read the entry from my senior scrapbook. Shaking my head free of the image, another one appeared of her walking away from Granddaddy's casket. She still walked with a limp. Guilt made me apprehensive about leaving her.

The next day, I felt better but I did not want to go with the others to Sea World. Raquel paying my entry for every theme park made me feel like a charity case. I told them I would stay in the hotel. A few hours after they left, I got a little stir crazy, my mind going a million miles a minute. Memories of the DECA competition from junior year and my life before the accident ran through my brain. I decided to venture out and try to find the same hotel where I stayed before. Walking the hotel strip, I remembered Shelly's senior class was supposed to be in Orlando for Spring Break. Maybe I would get a peek of some people I knew. I walked into a hotel and scanned the lobby, looking for anyone from North Charleston High. Suddenly, I caught a glimpse of myself in one of the lobby mirrors. The unrecognizable reflection shook me and I froze. It looked nothing like the confident, well put together teenage girl in high school. My face was hard. My posture was weak. My body was scarred and broken. I didn't want old friends or anyone else to see me like this. I ran out of the lobby as fast as I could, hoping no one saw me walking back to the motel. I sat in the dark room and waited for the others to return. Reality sank in. I was going back to Liberty Hill with no idea what to do. For six hours, I stared out the window as we drove to Charleston two days later. The driveway was empty when Raquel dropped me off at my mother's house. The Mazda was gone.

I spent the next few months racking my brain, trying to come up with a way to get back the future I lost. I considered another attempt at getting into the military. My first attempt was towards the end of my senior year, but the process stalled when I weighed in seven pounds too light. A second chance knocked on my door, months after losing the car. I told the handsome Marine recruiter about my unsuccessful attempt the year before. He suggested some strategies to gain weight and explained the benefits. The longer he stood in my mother's living room, the more I knew I was grasping at straws. Options were running out.

The last resort was my father. It was a long shot but I didn't know what else to do. Feeling hopeless with no money, I walked to his house in desperation on a September afternoon. I planned to present all the reasons he should help me. First, remind him how he wasn't there for me as a child. Mama could not do it anymore, so he had to step up. Fully intended to not leave empty-handed, I would demand hundreds of dollars in back child support. My emotions were on overdrive as I rehearsed what I was going to say. The absurdity of my plan did not occur to me while knocking on his door. Rose, his wife, let me in. I sat down with him and said everything I planned to say. Halfway through, tears fell from my eyes hearing how crazy I sounded. Still committed, I made my demands.

"I don't have any money," he said.

His words made me feel like such a fool. There was no way he would give me any money after the messages I left a year ago. Still, I assumed he would see my pain and try to help. Asking for money was easier than asking him to be the parent I so desperately needed. He continued to deny he had anything to give me. I stayed determined.

201

"Well, I'm not leaving until you give me something," I said, crying uncontrollably.

He reached into his wallet and handed me a $20 bill. I didn't want to take it but I was completely broke. My pride was destroyed, taking the money. Trying to save face, I quoted a Bible verse through my tears. Before walking, I spent time looking for the right one to say if he didn't give me what I needed.

"You're gonna pay for how you treated me today. The Bible says, let no man trouble me for I bear in my body the marks of the Lord Jesus." I stood up. I tearfully stuttered through my words. "I'm God's child. You don't have to help me." I stormed out and cried all the way back to my mother's house.

Days began to blur into each other. My eyes opened in the morning with no reason to get out of bed. Last year, there was school and friends to ensure I took a little time to be a girl. A car got me out of the house and off The Hill. All of that was gone. Sometimes, Aunt Debbie let me use her car to go to church on Sunday mornings. I would sneak into the balcony to avoid being seen. The first year after the accident, I covered my pain with a forced smile, but not anymore. I was exhausted. The pain was too much and all I wanted to do was hide. I sat in church services, wondering why I was there. The routine seemed pointless, but I was still drawn to it. Questions racked my brain desperately needing answers. None came from the religious clichés of the pulpit or the congregation who cheered for me in triumph but ignored me in deep distress.

The life I imagined for myself was nowhere in sight. September's fall air suffocated me as I sat on my mother's back porch, facing the empty driveway. I thought about the days I drove the Mazda to Sunset Memorial Gardens where my grandparents were buried. The empty plot they purchased for Mama, next to theirs, appeared in the driveway as my legs sank into the crevices of the brick steps. The sounds of my mother moving around in the backyard reminded me of the awful scrapbook entry I read to her.

Guilt sank me deeper into the cracked stone. My body slowly slid off the first porch step to the next. I felt the brick scratching my arms and legs. I wanted to go into the hole I saw in the driveway, where everything was lost.

A glimpse of something out of the corner of my eye partially brought me back to the present. In front of my mother's house was a white truck. Daddy was sitting at the wheel, in the middle of the street looking directly at me. He was just sitting there. I saw his face. It looked like he was laughing at me. His eyes were dark like empty holes. I wanted to scream at him but I couldn't move. My heart screamed in my head.

"Please, just leave. Are you really getting pleasure out of this? Please. Go!"

Finally, the truck pulled off. I shifted my hand to lift myself and ran into the house to my room. Every ounce of strength was used to get down the hall. I clutched the edge of my dresser for support and sank to the floor, pulling my knees close. My hands were shaking. My mouth, shivering. I could hear my heart beating out of my chest. Staring at the carpet, I grabbed my head with my hands and began to rock.

"Please, please stop. I can't do this anymore. Please, please stop this." I pleaded. "I know you can hear me. You have to show me you're real. I'm tired. I can't take it anymore. I need help. Please, help me."

I sat on the floor, alone with my tears. Then, still staring at the carpet, I felt the warm, defined silhouette of air wrap itself around my folded frame. Tears flowed freely as I surrendered and allowed myself to be held. I was safe. I was deeply loved. And I heard, very clearly:

"I got you. I got you. Let's do this."

Liberation

I sat in the warmth of God's arms for hours into sunset. The blazing heat of Charleston summers did not compare to the ever-present silhouette I allowed to join with my innermost being. Some days, I felt Him more than others, but he was always there, going to bed and waking up with me. This was different from everything family and the church said growing up. There was a tangible quality to God, defying religious clichés. He was relational. I could be completely honest with Him. There was no need to hide anything because He knew everything already. He knew my anger led to bitterness over the last two years. Hatred for him in my darkest moments, reached his ears every time I spoke the words. He was in David's dorm room when I wanted revenge. God quietly took all of my painful strikes, patiently waiting for me to let Him love me.

Discovering God in this new way, opened my heart and ears but I still had questions. There were many "whys" to be answered. I was okay with getting the answers later because they were about the past. I was more concerned about the future. Days were clearer but still empty. With nothing to do, I ran more errands. Walks to the Piggly Wiggly to get groceries were enjoyable. Spending more time with my mother was still not easy. Having meals together was all I could handle. Slowly, I started to get more comfortable living in the house. I learned to live with the changes my mother made though I never got used to them.

Mama's car sat in the backyard reminding me of what I lost until Aunt Barbara sold it. I was very angry at first, holding on to the possibility of getting the Buick up and running again. It felt like she was putting up roadblocks to keep me on Liberty Hill. Pursuing a life outside of current circumstances was a betrayal to her. The desire to be a devoted daughter blurred what I saw for my future. Suddenly,

Trident Technical College looked like a viable option. I could get my Associate's Degree and transfer to the College of Charleston. Many others took the same path. Maybe, I could get a good job after the two-year degree. All these options made sense but none of them were right for me. I felt the pull to cross the tracks like a rope tied around my soul.

Frustration grew, knowing I was supposed to be somewhere but not knowing how to get there. My room felt smaller by the day. I continued going to Aunt Debbie's house regularly, always coming back to sleep in my own bed. Daily walks were essential to peaceful sanity. Sometimes, Willie joined me and I was reminded of our walks as a little girl. Time together was nice, but guidance was what I needed. Willie knew I required more than he could give, though he always gave his best. Sometimes his best meant sending me to someone else.

One day, during one of our strolls, Willie told me Auntie Liz was asking about me. She wanted me to come by her house the next Sunday. Willie made it sound more like a summons than an invitation. After church, I drove Aunt Debbie's car to Auntie Liz's house. I knocked on her door with no clue what to expect. She invited me in but said this would not take long.

"Is that your car?" she asked, pointing outside.

"No ma'am," I replied. "That's my Aunt Debbie's car."

"Oh, is that where you're staying now?"

I was a bit thrown. Willie told her something.

"Um, not anymore. I'm pretty much back at my mother's."

She looked at me. "Well," she gathered herself. "I didn't call you here for that. What's going on with your schooling? I mean, you gonna go back? Or, whatchu doing?"

Auntie Liz asking about college caught me off guard. I explained about the remaining balance.

"How much is it?" she asked.

"It's $2,588. But I have a scholarship that will cover $2,000 of it."

"So, once you pay the 500, you can go back?" She made it sound so simple.

"I mean, I would probably have to enroll again. But yeah, after the balance is paid, I can go back."

"Ok. Well, whatever we need to do to get you back in school, we need to do it. 'Cause you don't belong here. You belong in school."

I stood there listening in shock. Someone actually saw me. Someone saw who I was and who I was meant to be.

"So, you need to get a little job for now." Auntie Liz continued. "Get the money you need to go back to school and get out of here."

"Yes ma'am," I said.

"Let me know if I can help you. I ain't gonna promise I can do much, but I'll try if I can."

"Ok," I said.

I wanted to hug her, but I had never seen Auntie Liz show much affection. I just thanked her and left. Suddenly, I had direction and guidance. After taking the car back to Aunt Debbie, I walked back to my mother's house. Old dreams of going to a big university, wearing a pageant crown someday, and being in television and movies were reignited, strolling Liberty Hill streets. The last two years made me forget them altogether. I forgot I was a dreamer and that I dreamed big. Voices in my head said it was not okay to dream, but they were wrong. I lived in a neighborhood founded by dreamers. I just had to take one dream at a time.

In the basic plan Auntie Liz laid out for me, priority one was getting a job. I set my sights on the banks in downtown Charleston. The idea of working in one of those offices reminded me of the executives I watched on soap operas. It seemed glamorous and important. For weeks, I caught the bus downtown in my dressiest outfits from high school passing as business attire. I applied for several teller positions but with no luck. Then, I shifted gears to the hotels just across the tracks but received no callbacks. I was getting discouraged until a church member said she would be happy to interview me for a position in her store at Charles Towne Square Mall. The mall was walking distance from the house. Knowing a manager made it seem like a sure thing. I went to the interview and tried to leave a good impression.

When weeks passed without a phone call, I was crushed. If I could not get a job with a connection, how would I get a job with a stranger? Doubts about the plan began to fill my head but something in me wanted to fight. I needed help from the One who held me the day I needed the most. I wanted to hear straight from Him this time. I decided to write God a letter like the one I wrote to David. Laying across my bed, I grabbed a small, old notebook I used for chemistry class and started writing.

"October 10, 1996
Dear God,

I'm having a really hard time with this faith and patience thing. I know I'm supposed to wait on you, but each day gets harder and worse. I hope not, because I can't believe everything, I've been through, is for nothing. I have to believe you have something more for me..."

After baring my soul, I grabbed a Bible and briskly flipped through the pages. I needed a response.

Only a few minutes passed before coming across a letter written to Colossians. "Keep praying," they were told, "And watch in the same with thanksgiving." God responded to my letter with one of his own. They were not the words I wanted to hear but they were good suggestions. It gave me enough courage to make one last effort when Uncle Jerome took me with him to pick up something at the Montgomery Ward department store. He encouraged me to seek out a manager and be the smart young lady he knew me to be. Left alone in the aisle, I walked around nervously looking for anyone with a store badge. I spotted a well-dressed, light-skinned woman and anxiously approached her.

"Excuse me," I tried to smile. "Is there a manager available?"

"I'm a manager," she said.

The butterflies in my stomach went crazy. "Oh. I was wondering if you were hiring."

"Well, we're looking for Christmas help but," she looked at me suspiciously. "How old are you?"

"Nineteen," I answered.

"Have you worked before?"

"Yes, I used to work at Sun Gospel Records. Sam…"

"Oh, yes," she softened a little. "I know Sam."

She asked about my availability. I explained I would be walking to work so I preferred day shifts but could be flexible. She appreciated my honesty.

"What's your name?" she asked.

"Ruthenna Porterfield."

"I'm Kim."

We spoke for a few minutes. Kim told me to come back and see her on Monday morning, where I would do the paperwork then. Uncle Jerome caught up with me about ten minutes later. He walked out with his package. I walked out with a job.

Work started the next week. Kim kept me on board after the holiday season. I looked forward to walking across the tracks to my first legitimate job. Every paycheck had a purpose. I helped my mother pay the phone bill and made sure to cover Cole's weekly calls from prison. For five months I saved to pay the balance at UNC Charlotte. In April, I called the radio station to send my Miss WPAL scholarship money to the school. By spring I was ready to re-enroll for the upcoming 1997 fall semester. My awful academic performance followed me through the eighteen-month hiatus, placing me on academic probation. But, it was official. I was going back to school in August.

Preparing my mother for my departure was not as pressing as it was two years earlier. Most of the task-driven work was done. She cooked and cleaned regularly. Aunt Barbara took her to get groceries and run errands. Trusting her with large sums of money was still out of the question. Dishonest friends from her past took advantage of her diminished ability to reason. Her checking account was taking noticeable hits. The best course of action was putting her on a monthly cash allowance to keep her financial losses to a minimum.

Bitterness towards my mother was something I wanted to dissipate as well. Mama was gone and I was holding my mother, Sandra Smalls, responsible for it. An innocent question made me realize she was not to blame.

"Quala, you going to work today?" She asked on a bright, April morning.

I had grown accustomed to living in the house on constant defense, expecting everything she said to be an attack.

"Yes. Why?" I retorted so sharply, it made her recoil.

She shook her head explaining. "I just wanted you to eat before you go."

My mother tried to be caring and it was thrown back in her face. I hated the way I made her feel. So afraid to deal with her episodes, I forgot they were short periods of time that were separate from who she was. For our relationship to get better, I decided to stop being afraid. I also needed to stop romanticizing Mama to cover the real source of my grief. I was not mourning the relationship before the accident, though I still longed for it. I was mourning the life I planned if the accident had not happened at all.

Winter turned to spring, and I discovered a second chance at my future and the truce I longed for. The relationship would look quite different since it would be with a different person. My mother could not see me as the girl she raised. Those memories were gone. I chose to be satisfied with her seeing me, simply, as someone she loved. Loving her the way I loved my Mama was not possible, but I would love her with no expectations.

As the days of my departure drew near, I spent more time with my mother. I tried to have conversations with her during meals. On rare occasions, I would watch a movie with her in the den. She enjoyed praying so I asked to join her a few times. She truly cherished our family prayer meetings. Sometimes, we sang devotional songs. I loved to see her close her eyes and wave her hands. It gave me so much pleasure to give her some joy.

August came. My excitement about going back to UNC Charlotte was different from two years ago. It felt like a transition instead of running away. Two weeks before leaving, I planned a small college send-off shower to allow others to celebrate the departure. I robbed people who loved me and who I appreciated, of the joy of celebrating my high school graduation. This was my opportunity to give it back. Many of my aunts, including some on my stepfather's side, came to my mother's house with food and gifts to furnish my dorm room. My mother was there, and we acknowledged her birthday which was the next day. The shower was a success.

I worked at the department store for one more week. Some co-workers gave me farewell gifts. Kim wrote me a glowing recommendation letter to give to prospective employers after I got settled at school. She was more than my manager by the time I left. She gave me a ride home when I worked night shifts, generously offering advice during the drive. As my superior, she corrected my mistakes and firmly called out inappropriate job behavior. Kim was my professional mentor. Saying goodbye to her was tearful.

Finally, the time came to leave. There weren't any tears on the morning of my departure. I was confident in my mother's ability to live independently and all the help she would receive. We ate breakfast together and said one last prayer. Uncle Jerome and my younger cousin, Sharel, backed into the empty driveway. My mother was not going on this trip. She sat aside while we placed my suitcases, my grandparents' old footlocker, and the TV I bought from my job into my uncle's truck. I went back into the house while my uncle secured everything.

"Ok. I think that's it," I said. "We're getting ready to pull out."

"Alright," my mother said. She walked with me to the door.

Uncle Jerome and Sharel were getting into the truck. "You ready Quala?" my uncle asked.

"Yep. I'm coming."

I gave my mother a sincere hug. "I love you," I said quickly. "I'll call you when we get there."

"I love you too," my mother said, hugging me back.

A smile lit her face as I walked out the door. I got in the truck and we pulled off. We crossed the railroad tracks and headed to Charlotte, North Carolina.

The three-hour drive went by fast. Uncle Jerome and Sharel helped me unpack and immediately got back on the road. My roommate came in soon after they left. We introduced ourselves. She told me she was from Charlotte. We talked about why she chose a school so close to home. As I listened to her and others I met, I learned everyone has a story. They are filled with moments we treasure and moments that shape us. Where we come from is part of our story. My roommate looked at me when she finished hers.

"So, where are you from?" she asked.

I looked at her and proudly said, "I'm from North Charleston, South Carolina. I grew up in a little neighborhood called Liberty Hill."

THE END

Works Cited

Blakeney, Barney. 2019. "Liberty Hill- One of North Charleston's
    Oldest Communities Being Polished For A Bright Future."
    The Charleston Chronicle, December 20.

The Charleston Chronicle. 2019. *Embracing The Liberty Hill
    Connection: Faith, Family and Community.* Charleston,
    September 28.

Acknowledgements

The first person who told me to write a book was a woman I worked with for only three months. Thank you, Erin Hawkins, for encouraging me to tell my story. It always begins with a seed.

But to grow, a seed needs consistent water. For years, as it lay under the dark soil of trying times, Tracey Reddick, you never allowed me to forget about this dream. "What about the book?" You would ask. "How's the book coming?" Your consistent persistence helped this book sprout in the darkness.

Finally, after breaking through the surface, the book needed a lot of light to fully bloom. Thank you, Dara Odeeyo, for challenging and upgrading my writing skill. Most of all, to my publisher, Brittney Holmes Jackson, and your entire team, thank you for your dedication to serving authors. I will always be grateful for your commitment to excellence, introducing me to literary legacy and ensuring this project lives on beyond the page.

COMING SOON

Things I Learned From Mama...After She Died

Follow the book journey at www.ruthennaporterfield.com